EOSINOPHILS, ALLERGY AND ASTHMA

Eosinophils, Allergy and Asthma

Edited by

A.B. KAY

Professor and Director,
Department of Allergy
and Clinical Immunology,
The National Heart
and Lung Institute,
London

BLACKWELL SCIENTIFIC PUBLICATIONS

OXFORD LONDON EDINBURGH

BOSTON MELBOURNE

Editorial Offices:
Osney Mead, Oxford OX2 0EL
25 John Street, London WC1N 2BL
23 Ainslie Place, Edinburgh EH3 6AJ
3 Cambridge Center, Suite 208
Cambridge, Massachusetts 02142, USA
54 University Street, Carlton
Victoria 3053, Australia

First published 1990

Photoset by Enset (Photosetting), Midsomer Norton, Bath, Avon

Printed and bound in Great Britain by Hartnolls Ltd, Bodmin, Cornwall

DISTRIBUTORS

Marston Book Services Ltd
PO Box 87
Oxford OX2 0DT
(*Orders:* Tel: 0865 791155
Fax: 0865 791927
Telex: 837515)

USA
Year Book Medical Publishers
200 North LaSalle Street
Chicago, Illinois 60601
(*Orders:* Tel: (312) 726-9733)

Canada
The C.V. Mosby Company
5240 Finch Avenue East
Scarborough, Ontario
(*Orders:* Tel: (416) 298-1588)

Australia
Blackwell Scientific Publications
(Australia) Pty Ltd
54 University Street
Carlton, Victoria 3053
(*Orders:* Tel: (03) 347-0300)

British Library
Cataloguing in Publication Data

Eosinophils, allergy and asthma.
1 Man. Blood. Eosinophils
I. Kay, A.B. (A. Barry)
612'.112
ISBN 0-632-02848-3

Contents

List of contributors

Catherine L. Akerman *Immunopharmacology Group, Clinical Pharmacology and Medicine I, Southampton General Hospital, Southampton SO9 4XY, UK.*

J.-C. Ameisen *Centre d'Immunologie et de Biologie Parasitaire, Unité Mixte INSERM, U167-CNRS624 Institut Pasteur, 59019 Lille, France.*

R.C. Baker *Beecham Pharmaceuticals, Research Division, Yew Tree Bottom Road, Epsom, Surrey KT18 5XQ, UK.*

R.L. Barker *Department of Immunology and the Division of Allergic Diseases and Internal Medicine, Mayo Clinic and Mayo Foundation, Rochester, Minnesota 55905, USA.*

P.J. Barnes *Department of Thoracic Medicine, National Heart and Lung Institute, Dovehouse Street, London SW3 6LY, UK.*

P. Braquet *I.H.B. Research Laboratories, 17 avenue Descartes, 92350 Le Plessis Robinson, France.*

A.E. Butterworth *Molteno Laboratories of Parasitology, Department of Pathology, University of Cambridge, Tennis Court Road, Cambridge CB2 1QP, UK.*

A. Capron *Centre d'Immunologie et de Biologie Parasitaire, Unité Mixte INSERM, U167-CNRS624 Institut Pasteur, 59019 Lille, France.*

Monique Capron *Centre d'Immunologie et de Biologie Parasitaire, Unité Mixte INSERM, U167-CNRS624 Institut Pasteur, 59019 Lille, France.*

Marie Carlson *The Laboratory for Inflammation Research, Department of Clinical Chemistry, University Hospital, S-751 85 Uppsala, Sweden.*

I.D. Chapman *Preclinical Research, Sandoz Ltd, CH-4002 Basel, Switzerland.*

K.F. Chung *Department of Thoracic Medicine, National Heart and Lung Institute, Dovehouse Street, London SW3 6LY, UK.*

M.K. Church *Immunopharmacology Group, Clinical Pharmacology and Medicine I, Southampton General Hospital, Southampton SO9 4XY, UK.*

Elaine J. Clutterbuck *National Institute for Medical Research, The Ridgeway, Mill Hill, London NW7 1AA, UK.*

R.M. Cook *Beecham Pharmaceuticals, Research Division, Yew Tree Bottom Road, Epsom, Surrey KT18 5XQ, UK.*

G. Dent *Department of Thoracic Medicine, National Heart and Lung Institute, Dovehouse Street, London SW3 6LY, UK.*

Christine De Vos *UCB Pharmaceutical Sector, Research and Development, Chemin du Foriest, B-1420 Braine-l'Alleud, Belgium.*

S.R. Durham *Department of Allergy and Clinical Immunology, National Heart and Lung Institute, Dovehouse Street, London SW3 6LY, UK.*

A. Etienne *I.H.B. Research Laboratories, 17 avenue Descartes, 92350 Le Plessis Robinson, France.*

A.J. Frew *Department of Allergy and Clinical Immunology, National Heart and Lung Institute, Dovehouse Street, London SW3 6LY, UK.*

G.J. Gleich *Department of Immunology and the Division of Allergic Diseases and Internal Medicine, Mayo Clinic and Mayo Foundation, Rochester, Minnesota 55905, USA.*

Adele Hartnell *Department of Allergy and Clinical Immunology, National Heart and Lung Institute, Dovehouse Street, London SW3 6LY, UK.*

Pat A. Hatt *Beecham Pharmaceuticals, Research Division, Yew Tree Bottom Road, Epsom, Surrey KT18 5XQ, UK.*

E. Hénocq *Unité de Pharmacologie cellulaire, Institut Pasteur, 25 Rue du Dr Roux, 75015 Paris, and 38 rue Beaujon, 75008 Paris, France.*

S.T. Holgate *Immunopharmacology Group, Clinical Pharmacology and Medicine I, Southampton General Hospital, Southampton SO9 4XY, UK.*

D. Hosford *I.H.B. Research Laboratories, 17 avenue Descartes, 92350 Le Plessis Robinson, France.*

Caroline J. Howell *Department of Allergy and Allied Respiratory Disorders, 4th Floor, Hunt's House, Guy's Hospital, London SE1 9RT, UK.*

Penny A. Hutson *Immunopharmacology Group, Clinical Pharmacology and Medicine I, Southampton General Hospital, Southampton SO9 4XY, UK.*

A.B. Kay *Department of Allergy and Clinical Immunology, National Heart and Lung Institute, Dovehouse Street, London SW3 6LY, UK.*

C. Kroegel *Department of Thoracic Medicine, National Heart and Lung Institute, Dovehouse Street, London SW3 6LY, UK.*

K. Kurihara *Department of Allergy and Clinical Immunology, National Heart and Lung Institute, Dovehouse Street, London SW3 6LY, UK.*

Sarah M. Laycock *Beecham Pharmaceuticals, Research Division, Yew Tree Bottom Road, Epsom, Surrey KT18 5XQ, UK.*

T.H. Lee *Department of Allergy and Allied Respiratory Disorders, 4th Floor, Hunt's House, Guy's Hospital, London SE1 9RT, UK.*

D.A. Loegering *Department of Immunology and the Division of Allergic Diseases and Internal Medicine, Mayo Clinic and Mayo Foundation, Rochester, Minnesota 55905, USA.*

A.J. MacDonald *Department of Allergy and Clinical Immunology, National Heart and Lung Institute, Dovehouse Street, London SW3 6LY, UK.*

D.J. McKean *Department of Immunology and the Division of Allergic Diseases and Internal Medicine, Mayo Clinic and Mayo Foundation, Rochester, Minnesota 55905, USA.*

R. Moqbel *Department of Allergy and Clinical Immunology, National Heart and Lung Institute, Dovehouse Street, London SW3 6LY, UK.*

J. Morley *Preclinical Research, Sandoz Ltd, CH-4002 Basel, Switzerland.*

N.R.J. Musgrove *Beecham Pharmaceuticals, Research Division, Yew Tree Bottom Road, Epsom, Surrey KT18 5XQ, UK.*

L.R. Pease *Department of Immunology and the Division of Allergic Diseases and Internal Medicine, Mayo Clinic and Mayo Foundation, Rochester, Minnesota 55905, USA.*

L. Prin *Centre d'Immunologie et de Biologie Parasitaire, Unité Mixte INSERM, U167-CNRS624 Institut Pasteur, 590109 Lille, France.*

B.A. Richardson *Molteno Laboratories of Parasitology, Department of Pathology, University of Cambridge, Tennis Court Road, Cambridge CB2 1QP, UK.*

S. Janet Rimmer *Immunopharmacology Group, Clinical Pharmacology and Medicine I, Southampton General Hospital, Southampton SO9 4XY, UK.*

C.J. Sanderson *National Institute for Medical Research, The Ridgeway, Mill Hill, London NW7 1AA, UK.*

H. Smith *Beecham Pharmaceuticals, Research Division, Yew Tree Bottom Road, Epsom, Surrey KT18 5XQ, UK.*

Janis K. Shute *Immunopharmacology Group, Clinical Pharmacology and Medicine I, Southampton General Hospital, Southampton SO9 4XY, UK.*

C. Soulard *I.H.B. Research Laboratories, 17 avenue Descartes, 92350 Le Plessis Robinson, France.*

Barbara A. Spicer *Beecham Pharmaceuticals, Research Division, Yew Tree Bottom Road, Epsom, Surrey KT18 5XQ, UK.*

R.M. Ten *Department of Immunology and the Division of Allergic Diseases and Internal Medicine, Mayo Clinic and Mayo Foundation, Rochester, Minnesota 55905, USA.*

F. Thonier *I.H.B. Research Laboratories, 17 avenue Descartes, 92350 Le Plessis Robinson, France.*

Kareen J.I. Thorne *Molteno Laboratories of Parasitology, Department of Pathology, University of Cambridge, Tennis Court Road, Cambridge CB2 1QP, UK.*

B.B. Vargaftig *Unité de Pharmacologie cellulaire, Institut Pasteur, 25 Rue du Dr Roux, 75015 Paris, France.*

P. Venge *The Laboratory for Inflammation Research, Department of Clinical Chemistry, University Hospital, S-751 85 Uppsala, Sweden.*

G.M. Walsh *Department of Allergy and Clinical Immunology, National Heart and Lung Institute, Dovehouse Street, London SW3 6LY, UK.*

T.L. Wasmoen *Department of Immunology and the Division of Allergic Diseases and Internal Medicine, Mayo Clinic and Mayo Foundation, Rochester, Minnesota 55905, USA.*

T. Yukawa *Department of Thoracic Medicine, National Heart and Lung Institute, Dovehouse Street, London SW3 6LY, UK.*

Preface

Eosinophil leucocytes continue to be a source of fascination and the subject of intensive research both by clinicians and scientists. Over the past few years there has been compelling evidence to implicate eosinophils in many of the inflammatory changes characteristic of atopic allergy and asthma. Although this broad hypothesis has not yet been proven, it is sufficiently persuasive for many groups within the pharmaceutical industry to direct their efforts identifying molecular targets associated with eosinophils and their products.

The present volume represents a summary of a 2-day meeting of 'Eosinophils, Allergy and Asthma' which was held at the Royal Society of Medicine, London, in December 1988. Many of the chapters have been reviewed and updated since this time and so the contents are a reasonable summary of the state of the art at the time of going to press.

A number of basic and applied aspects of eosinophil biology are addressed. These include molecular biological studies of the eosinophil major basic protein and interleukin-5; the nature and functional significance of receptors for immunoglobulins and adhesion glycoproteins; interactions between eosinophils and other inflammatory cells in allergy and asthma; and in particular an account of studies relating to interactions between platelet-activating factor and the eosinophil. The volume also contains chapters on anti-allergic drugs including those that might have specific anti-eosinophil actions.

Only time will tell whether the eosinophil is in fact a key effector cell in allergic inflammation and particularly in producing the mucosal damage characteristic of bronchial asthma. The possibility that eosinophils serve some other role such as repair, or are merely innocent bystanders, must also be kept in mind. Notwithstanding, this volume has attempted to summarize many of the important growth areas of eosinophil biology and how this information is being harnessed in a practical way to develop new therapeutic strategies.

I am very grateful to Miss Jennifer Mitchell for providing expert and untiring editorial assistance.

A.B. KAY
London, 1990

1 · Structural analyses of amino acid sequence and cDNA nucleotide sequence of eosinophil granule major basic protein: prediction of a novel pro-MBP molecule

G.J. Gleich,* L.R. Pease, D.J. McKean, D.A. Loegering, T.L. Wasmoen, R.M. Ten and R.L. Barker

Introduction

The eosinophil granule major basic protein (MBP) is the sole proteinaceous constituent of the crystalloid cores of the guinea pig eosinophil granule and has been localized to the core of the human eosinophil granule [1]. This relatively low molecular weight, highly cationic protein possesses a wide range of biological activities and has been implicated in tissue damage associated with eosinophil infiltrates, most notably as a mediator of damage to the respiratory epithelium in asthma [2]. Major basic protein is also cytotoxic to a wide variety of parasites and it can induce histamine release from rat mast-cells and human basophils [3]. These observations suggest that MBP is involved in antiparasitic defence mechanisms and immune hypersensitivity reactions. A knowledge of the structural basis of these biological functions could enhance future therapeutic approaches to control these pathological conditions. To this end, we determined the amino acid sequence of MBP [4] and utilizing this information we have constructed oligonucleotide probes to identify the cDNA coding for MBP. Analyses of the cDNA indicate that MBP is translated as a pre-pro-protein and the properties of the pro-portion of the pro-MBP suggest that the pro-portion may mask the toxic effects of mature MBP and protect the eosinophil from damage while MBP is processed through the endoplasmic reticulum [5].

Biochemical and amino acid sequence analyses of human eosinophil granule MBP

Initial approaches to the amino acid sequence analysis of MBP were hampered by the poor solubility of the molecule and its tendency to polymerize. In addition, the large number of arginines and absence of methionine made many conventional sequencing strategies unusable. Amino acid sequence of MBP was ultimately achieved by analyses

Supported by grants AI 09728, AI 15231, AI 00706, HD 22924, RR 00585, CA 26297 and CA 42100 from the National Institutes of Health and from the Mayo Foundation.
*To whom correspondence should be addressed.

of: (1) the amino terminus of the intact protein which permitted determination of the sequence through residue 60; (2) five peptides generated by cyanogen bromide-induced cleavage at tryptophan residues; and (3) a peptide derived from acid cleavage of a single aspartic acid–glycine bond at residue 71. Human eosinophil granule MBP was purified by lysing isolated eosinophil granules [6,7] and separating the protein constituents by gel filtration over Sephadex G-50 [7]. This purification scheme yields a protein that migrates as a single band on one dimension sodium dodecyl sulphate–polyacrylamide gel electrophoresis (SDS-PAGE) [6,7]. When this MBP was chromatographed by C18 reverse phase–high performance liquid chromatography (RP-HPLC) a single peak eluted from the column. When this MBP was analysed by two-dimensional gel electrophoresis only a single spot was detected. Non-equilibrium pH gradient gel electrophoresis was used in the first dimension here because MBP migrated off the gel when conventional isoelectric focusing was used. Interestingly, in the non-equilibrium pH gel gradient electrophoresis system, MBP migrates in advance of cytochrome C. Cytochrome C has a pI of 10.6. Although the exact pI of MBP has not been determined experimentally, the amino acid sequence predicts it at 10.9.

In initial studies to determine the amino acid sequence of MBP, a single amino

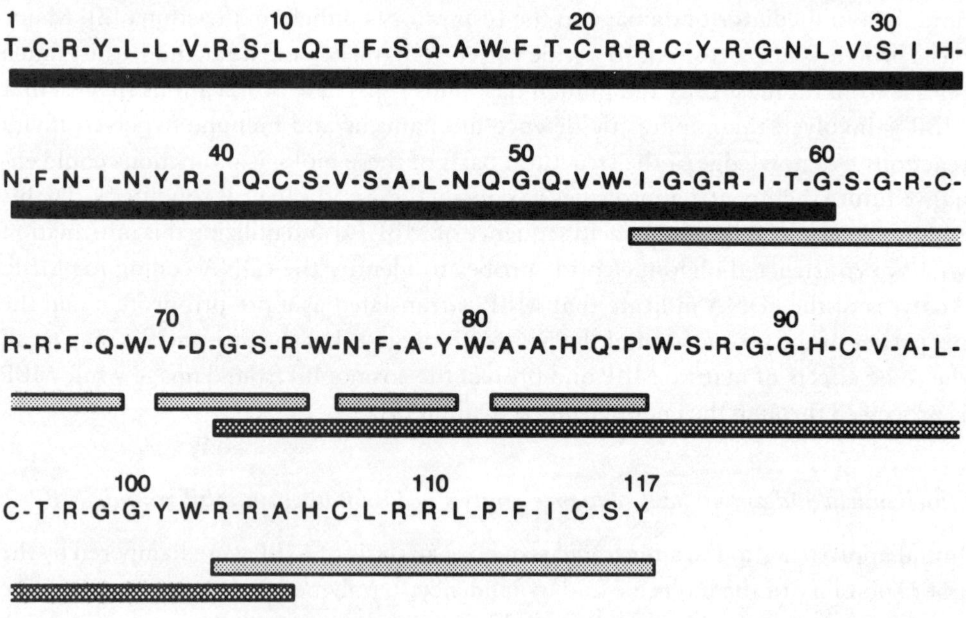

Fig. 1.1. Amino acid sequence of MBP. The amino acid sequence of MBP as determined from analyses of the intact protein and from isolated peptides. ■ Sequence obtained from N-terminal sequence of the intact protein. ▦ Sequence obtained from peptides generated by cleavage at tryptophan by cyanogen bromide. ▢ Sequence obtained from acetylation of the N-terminus, cleavage at aspartic acid in dilute acid, and analysis of the C-terminal peptide.

terminal sequence through residue 60 was found (Fig. 1.1). This sequence revealed a substantial number of arginines and the absence of any carboxylic acid-containing amino acids. The large number of arginine residues (17 in number for the complete protein) excluded trypsin as part of the sequencing strategy because the large number of tryptic peptides generated could not be resolved effectively. Also, many other conventional sequencing strategies were also unworkable because of the absence of critical amino acid residues such as methionine, glutamic acid and lysine. In addition, when the disulphide bonds were cleaved by reduction and alkylation of MBP in denaturing solvents, the resultant MBP was insoluble in most pH buffers.

The most useful method found to generate peptides from MBP was cleavage at tryptophan. Here, eight peptides were generated and all were isolated by RP-HPLC. Five of these peptides were purified to homogeneity and sequenced. Partial cleavage at tryptophan 69 provided two peptides, namely residues 54–68 and residues 54–75. The sequence of peptide 54–75 identified an aspartic residue at position 71. The favourable solubility of MBP at acid pH and the existence of only one aspartic acid residue at a critical location suggested that we could use dilute acid to cleave the aspartic acid–glycine bond at residue 71–72. Incubation of MBP at 105°C in 0.25 M acetic acid resolves the molecule into two peptides. The molecular weights of these peptides as determined by SDS-PAGE were 7250 and 4800. These weights correspond well to the theoretical peptides generated by cleavage at this bond. Analysis of the peptide mixture revealed a double amino acid sequence corresponding to the N-terminal sequence plus the sequence beginning at residue 72. However, attempts to separate these new peptides by RP-HPLC were unsuccessful. Therefore, the amino terminus of MBP was blocked by acetylation prior to the dilute acid cleavage so that only the sequence from residue 72 was detected. The resulting peptide mixture yielded a single amino acid sequence (residues 72–105, see Fig. 1.1), which allowed ordering of the carboxy terminal peptides generated by cleavage at tryptophan. We were repeatedly unable to sequence completely from residue 72 to 117 due to a precipitous loss in yield associated with cleavage of the histidine residue at position 83. Furthermore, attempts to confirm the carboxy terminal residue through the use of carboxypeptidase were unsuccessful.

Figure 1.1 shows the constituent peptides used to define the amino acid sequence of MBP. The molecular mass of MBP calculated from this sequence is 13 801 daltons and the predicted pI is 10.9. A homology search utilizing the National Biomedical Research Foundation database revealed that MBP has no significant primary sequence homology toward any known protein.

These analyses of the MBP amino acid sequence were complicated by the fact that MBP readily aggregates with itself and other proteins and at alkaline pH can only be isolated as a monomer after alkylation. Human MBP contains nine half-cystines and guinea pig MBP possesses two reactive sulphhydryl groups [8]. Measurements of the number of reactive sulphhydryls in human MBP indicate that more than two are present, but the rapidity of aggregation hampered attempts to determine the actual number. Also, as noted above, the nature of MBP precluded many conventional amino acid sequencing strategies. Nonetheless, the amino acid sequence of the intact protein yielded over half the total residues in the molecule, namely 60 residues. The remaining residues were defined by sequencing peptides generating cyanogen–bromide induced cleavage at tryptophans. The chemistry of this reaction is not well understood [9], but the cleavage occurs to the carboxyl side of tryptophan and modifies this residue so that it cannot be identified by conventional HPLC analysis of the phenylthiohydantoins. Incomplete cleavage at tryptophan position 69 resulted in a partial purified peptide containing residues 54–75 and this provided a critical overlap with the known amino terminal sequence and the remaining sequence. The identification of the aspartic acid–glycine bond at residue 71–72 and the ability to cleave this with acid enabled us to order the remaining residues of the carboxy terminal residue.

The marked basicity of MBP can be explained by the presence of 17 arginine residues and only one carboxylic acid-containing residue. MBP with a calculated pI of 10.9 thus is one of the most basic proteins known. The MBP sequence also contains numerous glycine and alanine residues, a high proportion of amino acids with apolar side chains, and a high fractional content of aromatic residues. This arrangement of high charge and apolar residues on the surface of MBP may be crucial to its biological functions. Indeed, the extreme charge in hydrophobic properties may be responsible for some of the biologic activities attributed to MBP including: interaction with coagulation factors [8], activation of mast cells and basophils [10,11], cytotoxicity [3,12,13] and toxicity for parasites [14–16]. A large number of neurotoxins and cytotoxins isolated from snakes are also highly cationic, relatively small ($M_r < 10\,000$) proteins. There are also many cationic peptides with marked cytotoxic properties such as melittin from bee venom [17], the pardaxins from the sole *Pardachirus pavoninus* [18] and mastoparans from wasp venom [19]. These peptides share cationic charge along with a marked number of hydrophobic residues. Melittin and the mastoparans are especially distinguished by periodicity of their hydrophobic residues, which describe an amphiphilic helix. The mechanism of their toxicity is not known, but all of the peptides bind to cell membranes and are able to promote cell fusion. Major basic protein has similar hydrophobic and cationic properties, but it is not predicted to have any amphiphilic helix segments. Nonetheless, regions of hydrophobicity of protein are clearly accessible and it is possible that the cationic charge serves to attract MBP to the negatively charged cell surface whereupon the apolar residues insert into and perturb the lipid milieu.

Nucleotide sequence of MBP cDNA

To identify the cDNA for MBP, mixed synthetic oligodeoxyribonucleotide probes were synthesized for residues 50–55 and 75–81. These gave degeneracies of 96- and

32-fold, respectively. Because MBP appears to be constitutively produced by HL-60 cells [20], we probed a lambda gt10 HL-60 cDNA library kindly provided by Dr David Bentley (ICRF Laboratories, London, England). The lambda gt10 HL-60 cDNA library was analysed by absorbing phage onto nylon membranes and exposing the denatured phage to the labelled oligodeoxyribonucleotide probes. Recombinant clones positive to both of the probes were selected from the library and plaque purified. The DNA from the recombinant phage was purified [21] and restricted with EcoR1 which yielded a single insert fragment of approximately 900 based pairs. This fragment was ligated into M13mp10 and sequenced by the dideoxy chain determination method [22].

The nucleotide sequence of human MBP is shown in Fig. 1.2. As is typical of many cDNAs, the nucleotide sequence of the isolated clone contains sequences similar to consensus sequence associated with eukaryotic initiation [23] and polyadenylation signals [24]. Primer extension reactions [25] utilizing purified HL-60 mRNA indicated that the MBP cDNA is the same length as full length message and therefore it contains the entire coding sequence of the protein.

The longest open reading frame of the nucleotide sequence codes for a protein of 220 amino acids including a terminal sequence of 117 amino acids, which is identical to the amino acid sequence of MBP (Fig. 1.1). However, the MBP sequence is preceded by a 15 amino acid putative signal peptide [26], which is typical of secreted proteins, and by a middle sequence of 90 amino acids; neither of these sequences are present in the mature protein. These data suggested that MBP is initially translated as a pre-pro-protein which is cotranslationally modified to pro-MBP and post-translationally modified to MBP.

Major basic protein has 17 strongly basic amino acids, only one strongly acidic amino acid and a predicted pI of 10.9. As shown in Table 1.1, the pro-portion of pro-MBP has 26 strongly acidic amino acids, seven strongly basic amino acids and a pI of 3.9. The combination of the acidic and basic peptides in pro-MBP has a slightly acidic pI of 6.2. Translation of MBP as a pro-protein may mask the toxic effects of mature MBP and protect the eosinophil from damage while the protein is processed through the endoplasmic reticulum. Heparin, an acidic mucopolysaccharide, reacts with MBP [8] and inhibits its toxicity [3,14] suggesting that MBP would be neutralized by an acidic precursor.

Several possibilities exist for the processing of the pro-MBP molecule. First, the acid portion could be cleaved during transport from the endoplasmic reticulum to the granule and toxic MBP could be stored in the granule. Second, the pro-MBP could be initially stored in the granule and subsequently processed to toxic MBP, which would then crystallize to form the granule core. Third, pro-MBP could crystallize during maturation and form the granule core; immediately before secretion pro-MBP would be further processed to the toxic form of MBP. Among these possibilities we favour the second one, namely the initial storage of pro-MBP in the granule followed by

```
                                    TER
  1 AAAAGAAGGAC CTG GGC TTT GGG AAG ATC TAA AGA CCC AGG AAG GTC TCT GGG TGG GAT AAA

-15              M   K   L   P   L   L   L   A   L   L   F   G   A   V   S   A   L   H
 63 GCC AAG ATG AAA CTC CCC CTA CTT CTG GCT CTT CTA TTT GGG GCA GTT TCT GCT CTT CAT
  4 L   R   S   E   T   S   T   F   E   T   P   L   G   A   K   T   L   P   E   D
123 CTA AGG TCT GAG ACT TCC ACC TTT GAG ACC CCT TTG GGT GCT AAG ACG CTG CCT GAG GAT
 24 E   E   T   P   E   Q   E   M   E   E   T   P   C   R   E   L   E   E   E   E
183 GAG GAG ACA CCA GAG CAG GAG ATG GAG GAG ACC CCT TGC AGG GAG CTG GAG GAA GAG GAG
 44 E   W   G   S   G   S   E   D   A   S   K   K   D   G   A   V   E   S   I   S
243 GAG TGG GGC TCT GGA AGT GAA GAT GCC TCC AAG AAA GAT GGG GCT GTT GAG TCT ATC TCA
 64 V   P   D   M   V   D   K   N   L   T   C   P   E   E   E   D   T   V   K   V
303 GTG CCA GAT ATG GTG GAC AAA AAC CTT ACG TGT CCT GAG GAA GAG GAC ACA GTA AAA GTG
                                *
 84 V   G   I   P   G   C   Q   T   C   R   Y   L   L   V   R   S   L   Q   T   F (13)
363 GTG GGC ATC CCT GGG TGC CAG ACC TGC CGC TAC CTC CTG GTG AGA AGT CTT CAG ACG TTT
104 S   Q   A   W   F   T   C  .R   R   C   Y   R   G   N   L   V   S   I   H   N (33)
423 AGT CAA GCT TGG TTT ACT TGC CGG AGG TGC TAC AGG GGC AAC CTG GTT TCC ATC CAC AAC
124 F   N   I   N   Y   R   I   Q   C   S   V   S   A   L   N   Q   G   Q   V   W (53)
483 TTC AAT ATT AAT TAT CGA ATC CAG TGT TCT GTC AGC GCG CTC AAC CAG GGT CAA GTC TGG
144 I   G   G   R   I   T   G   S   G   R   C   R   R   F   Q   W   V   D   G   S (73)
543 ATT GGA GGC AGG ATC ACA GGC TCG GGT CGC TGC AGA CGC TTT CAG TGG GTT GAC GGC AGC
164 R   W   N   F   A   Y   W   A   A   H   Q   P   W   S   R   G   G   H   C   V (93)
603 CGC TGG AAC TTT GCG TAC TGG GCT GCT CAC CAG CCC TGG TCC CGC GGT GGT CAC TGC GTG
184 A   L   C   T   R   G   G   Y   W   R   R   A   H   C   L   R   R   L   P   F (113)
663 GCC CTG TGT ACC CGA GGA GGC TAC TGG CGT CGA GCC CAC TGC CTC AGA AGA CTT CCT TTC
204 I   C   S   Y   TER                                                           (117)
723 ATC TGT TCC TAC TGA GCT GGT CCC AGC CAG CAG TTC AGA GCT GCC CTC TCC TGG GCA GCT
                                                           TER
783 GCC TCC CCT CCT CTG CTT GCC ATC CCT CCC TCC ACC TCC CTG CAA TAA AAT GGG TTT TAC
    TER
843 TGA AAA ...
```

Table 1.1. Approximate isoelectric points of MBP and BTAH derived from translation of their cDNA[a] sequences

Protein	Amino acids	Strongly basic amino acids (K,R)	Strongly acidic amino acids (D,E)	pI
Human MBP	117	17	1	10.9
pro-portion	90	7	26	3.9
pro	207	24	27	6.2
BTAH	45	10	0	9.6
pro-portion	64	3	11	3.6
pro	109	13	11	7.6

[a]Isoelectric points (pIs) calculated by Trans program (DNAstar, Inc., Madison, WI). BTAH–barley toxin α-hordothionin, MBP–major basic protein.

processing to toxic MBP and crystallization of toxic MBP to form the granule core. Our preference for this mechanism is based on several experimental observations. First, basophilic staining granules [27] are present in eosinophilic myocytes from the bone marrow, whereas mature eosinophils do not show basophilia suggesting that the cationicity of the granule increases as it develops. Second, prior studies of eosinophil granules [28] showed that lysis at pH 2 reduces granule turbidity by over 90% and liberates MBP; no evidence of a pro-MBP molecule was found. Third, SDS-PAGE of acid solubilized guinea pig granule crystalloid cores showed only a single band migrating with the molecular weight of toxic MBP [1]. Because virtually all of the core substance was solubilized in this latter experiment, this observation suggests that toxic MBP forms the granule crystalloid. Thus, these data are in keeping with the hypothesis that pro-MBP is initially sequestered in the granule and processed to toxic MBP, which is subsequently stored in the crystalloid.

To determine whether acidic precursors are unique to MBP or if it is found in other toxic proteins, the Genetic Sequence Data Bank and the Protein Identification Resource were searched. These results indicated that MBP shows little sequence homology with known genes and proteins. Collection of the cDNA sequences of toxic basic proteins from a literature search revealed that none of the reported cDNAs from basic toxins codes for an acidic precursor. However, the cDNA of barley toxin alpha-hordothionin [29] codes for a nearly neutral precursor. Interestingly, the pI profile of

Fig. 1.2. Nucleotide sequence of human MBP cDNA. Nucleotides 1–848 and amino acids 15–207 are numbered on the left of the figure. Eukaryotic initiation signal at position 64–71 and polyadenylation signal at position 826–831 are underlined. An arrow indicates putative signal peptide cleavage site. An asterisk indicates first amino acid in eosinophil granule MBP. Amino acids of eosinophil granule MBP are numbered in parentheses on the right of the figure. TER: termination.

the barley toxin alpha-hordothionin is surprisingly similar to MBP (Table 1.1). The pro-portion of pro-barley toxin alpha-hordothionin has 11 strongly acidic amino acids, three strongly basic amino acids and a pI of 3.6, whereas the toxin itself has 10 strongly basic amino acids, no acidic amino acids and a pI of 9.6; the pro-molecule has a pI of 7.6. In the barley toxin, the signal peptide is immediately followed by the mature protein and then by the acidic pro-portion. Barley toxin alpha-hordothionin is lysine and cysteine rich and comprises 4% of endosperm protein where it may be extrinsically associated with the endoplasmic reticulum [30]. Although thionins are orally innocuous, they are toxic to laboratory animals by intraperitoneal injection, as well as to cultured mammalian cells, yeast and phytopathogenic bacteria [29]. Thionins modified cell membrane permeability and induced a rapid leakage of ions and low molecular weight compounds, which may be responsible for the inhibition of protein and nucleic acid synthesis by thionins [31]. A function for the pro-portion of the barley toxin has not been suggested [29]; one possibility is that the acidic pro-portion of the barley toxin may neutralize the basic mature protein, as we have already suggested for the precursor of MBP and that this mechanism may be found in other cells which produce cationic toxins which damage cell membranes.

Summary

The amino acid sequence and the cDNA nucleotide sequence of eosinophil granule MBP have been determined. The amino acid sequence of MBP was complicated by the marked tendency of MBP to polymerize and by the absence of critical residues such as methionine, lysine, and glutamic acid, as well as by the large number of arginine residues precluding the use of trypsin. However, cyanogen-bromide induced cleavage at tryptophan and acid-induced cleavage at aspartic acid were used successfully to obtain peptides permitting a definition of the amino acid sequence of MBP. Knowledge of the amino acid sequence permitted construction of mixed synthetic oligodeoxyribonucleotide probes for MBP and identification of MBP cDNA from a HL-60 cDNA library. The nucleotide sequence of MBP cDNA indicates that MBP is translated as a 25.2 kD pre-pro-protein. The 9.9-kD pro-portion of pro-MBP is rich in glutamic acid and has a calculated pI of 3.9 while pro-MBP has a calculated pI of 6.2. These results suggest that MBP is translated as a non-toxic precursor which protects the eosinophil from damage, while the protein is being processed through the endoplasmic reticulum to its sequestered site in the granule core as toxic MBP. Analysis of literature suggests that other cationic proteins which are able to damage cell membranes may also be processed from non-toxic precursors containing distinct anionic and cationic regions.

References

1 Lewis DM, Lewis JC, Loegering DA, Gleich GJ. Localization of the guinea pig eosinophil major basic protein to the core of the granule. *J. Cell Biol.* 1978;77:702.

2 Frigas E, Gleich GJ. The eosinophil and the pathophysiology of asthma. *J. Allergy Clin. Immunol.* 1986;77:527.

3 Gleich GJ, Adolphson CR. The eosinophilic leukocyte: structure and function. *Adv. Immunol.* 1986;**39**:177–253.

4 Wasmoen TL, Bell MP, Loegering DA, Gleich GJ, Prendergast FG, McKean DJ. Biochemical and amino acid sequence analysis of human eosinophil granule major basic protein. *J. Biol. Chem.* 1988;**263**:12559.

5 Barker RL, Gleich GJ, Pease LR. Acidic precursor revealed in human eosinophil granule major basic protein cDNA. *J. Exp. Med.* 1988;**168**:1493.

6 Gleich GJ, Loegering DA, Mann KG, Maldonado JE. Comparative properties of the Charcot-Leyden crystal protein and the major basic protein from human eosinophils. *J. Clin. Invest.* 1976;**57**:633.

7 Slifman NR, Loegering DA, McKean DJ, Gleich GJ. Ribonuclease activity associated with human eosinophil-derived neurotoxin and eosinophil cationic protein. *J. Immunol.* 1986;**137**:2913.

8 Gleich GJ, Loegering DA, Kueppers F, Bajaj SP, Mann KG. Physiochemical and biological properties of the major basic protein from guinea pig eosinophil granules. *J. Exp. Med.* 1974;**140**:313.

9 Huang HV, Bond MW, Hunkapiller MW, Hood LE. Cleavage at tryptophanyl residues with dimethyl sulfoxide-hydrochloric acid and cyanogen bromide. *Methods Enzymol.* 1983;**91**:318–324.

10 O'Donnell MC, Ackerman SJ, Gleich GJ, Thomas LL. Activation of basophil and mast cell histamine release by eosinophil granule major basic protein. *J. Exp. Med.* 1983;**157**:1981.

11 Zheutlin LM, Ackerman SJ, Gleich GJ, Thomas LL. Stimulation of basophil and rat mast cell histamine release by eosinophil granule-derived cationic proteins. *J. Immunol.* 1984;**133**:2180.

12 Gleich GJ, Frigas E, Loegering DA, Wassom DL, Steinmuller D. Cytotoxic properties of the eosinophil major basic protein. *J. Immunol.* 1979;**123**:2925.

13 Frigas E, Loegering DA, Gleich GJ. Cytotoxic effects of the guinea pig eosinophil major basic protein on tracheal epithelium. *Lab. Invest.* 1980;**42**:35.

14 Butterworth AE, Wassom DL, Gleich GJ, Loegering DA, David JR. Damage to schistosomula of *Schistosoma mansoni* induced directly by eosinophil major basic protein. *J. Immunol.* 1979;**122**:221.

15 Wassom DL, Gleich GJ. Damage to *Trichinella spiralis* newborn larvae by eosinophil major basic protein. *Am. J. Trop. Med. Hyg.* 1979;**28**:860.

16 Kierszenbaum F, Ackerman SJ, Gleich GJ. Destruction of bloodstream forms of *Trypanosoma cruzi* by eosinophil granule major basic protein. *Am. J. Trop. Med. Hyg.* 1981;**30**:775.

17 Schroder E, Lubke K, Lehmann M, Beetz I. Haemolytic activity and action on the surface tension of aqueous solutions of synthetic melittins and their derivatives. *Experientia (Basel)* 1971;**27**:764–765.

18 Thompson SA, Tachibana K, Nakanishi K, Kubota I. Melittin-like peptides from the shark-repelling defense secretion of the sole *Pardachinus pavoninus*. *Science* 1986;**233**:341.

19 Hopp TA, Woods KR. Prediction of protein antigenic determinants from amino acid sequences. *Proc. Natl. Acad. Sci. USA* 1981;**78**:3824–3828.

20 Fischkoff SA, Pollak A, Gleich GJ, Testa JR, Misawa S, Reber TJ. Eosinophilic differentiation of the human promyelocytic leukemia cell line, HL-60. *J. Exp. Med.* 1984;**160**:179.

21 Yamamoto KR, Alberts BM, Benzinger R, Lawhorne L, Treiber G. Rapid bacteriophage sedimentation in the presence of polyethylene glycol and its application to large-scale virus purification. *Virology* 1970;**40**:734.

22 Biggin MD, Gibson TJ, Hong GF. Buffer gradient gels and ^{35}S label as an aid to rapid DNA sequence determination. *Proc. Natl. Acad. Sci. USA* 1983;**80**:3963.

23 Kozak M. Compilation and analysis of sequences upstream from the translational start site in eukaryotic mRNAs. *Nucleic Acid Res.* 1984;**12**:857.

24 Proudfoot NJ, Brownlee GG. 3′ non-coding region sequences in eukaryotic messenger RNA. *Nature (Lond)* 1975;**263**:211.

25 Geliebter J, Zeff RA, Melvold RW, Nathenson SG. Mitotic recombination in germ cells generated two major histocompatibility complex mutant genes shown to be identical by RNA sequence analysis: Kbm9 and Kbm6. *Proc. Natl. Acad. Sci. USA* 1986;**83**:3371.

26 von Heijne G. Patterns of amino acids near signal-sequence cleavage sites. *Eur. J. Biochem.* 1983;**133**:17.

27 Ackerman GA. Eosinophilic leukemia: a morphologic and histochemical study. *Blood* 1964;**24**:372.

28 Gleich GJ, Loegering DA, Maldonado JE. Identification of a major basic protein in guinea pig eosinophil granules. *J. Exp. Med.* 1973;**137**:1459.

29 Ponz F, Paz-Ares J, Hernandez-Lucas C, Garcia-Olmedo F, Carbonero P. Cloning and nucleotide sequence of a cDNA encoding the precursor of the barley toxin alpha-hordothionin. *Eur. J. Biochem.* 1986;**156**:131.

30 Ponz F, Paz-Ares J, Hernandez-Lucas C, Carbonero P, Garcia-Olmedo F. Synthesis and processing of thionin precursors in developing endosperm from barley (*Hordeum vulgare* L.). *Embo J.* 1985;**2**:1035.

31 Carrasco L, Vazquez D, Hernandez-Lucas C, Carbonero P, Garcia-Olmedo F. Thionins: Plant peptides that modify membrane permeability in cultured mammalian cells. *Eur. J. Biochem.* 1981;**116**:185.

2 · Immunoglobulin receptors on eosinophil leucocytes

Monique Capron,* L. Prin, J.-C. Ameisen and A. Capron

Summary

Human eosinophils possess membrane receptors for immunoglobulins (IgG, IgE, IgA and probably IgM), which in addition to complement receptors (CR1 and CR3) allow them to interact with immunoglobulins, antigens and immune complexes. The IgG receptor is distinct from the neutrophil IgG receptor, and its expression is increased by chemotactic factors. The main characteristics of IgE receptor (FcεRII) are summarized and the comparison between eosinophil and B cell FcεRII (or CD23) reveals the existence of a common structure. Binding of IgA to activated eosinophils by using flow cytofluorometry and binding assays is reported. Pharmacologically active mediators eosinophil peroxidase (EPO), major basic protein (MBP) leukotriene (LT) C_4 and platelet-activating factor (PAF)-acether can be released after immunoglobulin-dependent stimulation. A differential release of eosinophil mediators in response to IgE versus IgG-dependent stimulation is reported, and illustrated by electron microscopy studies on tissue eosinophils. Finally, the effects of some drugs (cetirizine, disodium cromoglycate and PAF-antagonists) on the different steps of eosinophil activation tend to support the hypothesis of selectivity of mediator release. Taken all together, these results might have significant implications in the understanding of the physiopathology of allergic reactions, but also in the definition of novel therapeutic strategies.

Introduction

Identified at the end of the 19th century, eosinophils have been considered for a long time as 'inflammatory cells', able to be mobilized at the sites of inflammation by various chemotactic factors. Increased blood eosinophilia has been associated mainly with parasitic and allergic diseases, and much of our knowledge on eosinophil function in human pathology derives from studies performed in parasitic infections or in allergic diseases during the last decade. Evidence [1] indicates the 'dual' function of eosinophils: eosinophils are involved in protection, both by their down-regulatory

This work was supported by the Unité Mixte INSERM U167-CNRS 624, Institut Pasteur, Lille, France.
*To whom correspondence should be addressed.

effect of immediate-type hypersensitivity reactions and by their cytotoxic role against parasite larvae. However the identification of eosinophil cytolytic molecules and their involvement in damage of normal mammalian cells conferred to eosinophils a role in pathology. Finally the demonstration of membrane receptors for IgE and their participation in the release of mediators suggested the essential role of eosinophils in hypersensitivity reactions.

After a brief survey of some general aspects concerning eosinophil membrane receptors, the release of pharmacologically active mediators will be discussed in response to immunoglobulin-dependent activation. Some new therapeutic approaches will then be considered in this context.

General aspects

Similar to other leucocytes, eosinophils possess membrane receptors for IgG (FcγR) for IgE (FcεR) and, more recently described, for IgA (FcαR), whereas the existence of receptors for IgM has also been suspected. Besides these Fc receptors, eosinophils have receptors for C3b (CR1) and for C3bi (CR3) allowing them to interact with immunoglobulins, antigens and immune complexes. The presence of pharmacological receptors has also been demonstrated, for oestradiol, histamine, glucocorticoids and more recently PAF-acether.

Eosinophils can be incriminated in diseases by releasing various preformed mediators, including specific components such as the granule cationic proteins, major basic protein (MBP) present in the crystalloid, eosinophil cationic protein (ECP), eosinophil-derived neurotoxin (EDN), eosinophil peroxidase (EPO), present in the matrix. Eosinophils can also generate newly formed mediators such as prostaglandins (PGE_2), leukotrienes (LTC_4 5- or 15-HETE) or PAF-acether. Eosinophils from hypereosinophilic patients (with helminth infections, allergic diseases, with the hypereosinophilic syndrome (HES), or with some myeloproliferative disorders) are very heterogeneous, with respect to their morphology, membrane receptors or oxida-

Table 2.1. Heterogeneity of human eosinophils

	Normodense	Hypodense
Presence	Normal subjects, low eosinophilia	High hypereosinophilia tissues
Density on metrizamide	High ($d > 1.130$)	Low ($d < 1.126$)
Granules	Electrondense crystalloid, radiolucent matrix	Reduced size; Loss of electron density; Heterogeneity
Nucleus		Polysegmented
Oxidative metabolism	High	Impaired
Membrane receptors		Increased FcεRII & CR3
Antiparasite cytotoxicity	IgG-dependent	IgE-dependent

tive metabolism. By centrifugation upon discontinuous density gradients, two subpopulations of human eosinophils differing by their cell density ('normodense' or 'hypodense') and by their morphology (inversion of the electron density of the crystalloid and reduced size of the granules in the case of hypodense eosinophils) were identified. Hypodense eosinophils represent not only the activated state but also the cells in contact to the target tissues, directly involved in pathology. The main characteristics allowing to differentiate hypodense and normodense eosinophils are summarized in Table 2.1.

Immunoglobulin receptors

Receptors for IgG

Since human IgG antibodies have represented the first immunoglobulin class to be involved in eosinophil-mediated killing of schistosomula [2], the receptor for IgG was the first Fc receptor identified on the membrane of human eosinophils. Whereas the first reports have concerned heterologous systems using animal immunoglobulins, more recent studies on the binding of human IgG to human eosinophils were performed. In summary, by a rosette assay, the receptor for IgG binds to the four IgG isotypes without distinct specificity [3] but it is likely that the affinity for the different subclasses might vary, as shown for rat IgG2a and IgG2c [4]. This is suggested by analysis of IgG cytophilically bound to human eosinophils *in vivo*: very few cytophilic IgG are detected after addition of total anti-IgG antibodies [5], in contrast to the presence of cytophilically bound IgG4 revealed by the addition of anti-IgG4 [M. Capron, unpublished results]. The molecular weight of human eosinophil IgG receptor is different from the neutrophil IgG receptor (43 kD versus 52–68 kD) and their binding affinity for the various IgG subclasses seems distinct [6]. Further studies are needed to classify human eosinophil IgG receptor in the family of FcγRII or FcγRIII, for instance, by using monoclonal antibodies or cDNA probes now available. Eosinophil FcγR is inducible as suggested by its increased expression after incubation with various soluble factors *in vitro*, including chemotactic factors such as eosinophil chemotactic factor of anaphylaxis or ECF-A (7), formyl-methionyl-leucyl-phenylalanine (FMLP) or LTB_4 [8].

Receptors for IgE

IgE receptors have been demonstrated on human eosinophils and they participate directly in the effector function of eosinophils against parasite larvae. The main characteristics of eosinophil IgE receptors are summarized in Table 2.2 and reviewed in detail in reference [9]. The production of a monoclonal antibody (BB10) raised against human FcεR-positive eosinophils and able to inhibit the IgE-dependent

Table 2.2. IgE receptors on human eosinophils

Detection on a subpopulation of eosinophils
Increased expression in hypereosinophilic patients
Involved in cytotoxicity against parasites (hypodense)
Low affinity for IgE monomers (10^7 M^{-1})
Common antigenicity with FcεR of B-cells, platelets and monocytes (FcεRII)

cytotoxicity of eosinophils, platelets and monocytes, has confirmed the common antigenicity of these FcεR, now referred to as FcεRII [10].

A common feature of these FcεRII is their increased expression on activated cells. In the particular situation of human eosinophils, IgE-dependent effector function seems to be restricted to a subpopulation of eosinophils with low density (hypodense), suggesting that the presence of a functional FcεR could be considered as one marker of eosinophil heterogeneity. Another membrane receptor (CR3) which acts in synergy with FcεRII has also an increased expression on hypodense eosinophils [11]. Eosinophil heterogeneity was confirmed by using the monoclonal antibody (mAb) BB10, which selectively stains hypodense and not normodense eosinophils [10]. In addition, this mAb allowed us to biochemically characterize the eosinophil receptor for IgE, by using immunosorbent chromatography of eosinophil detergent extracts, passed over either IgE or BB10 immunosorbents [12]. Under reducing conditions, three polypeptide fragments were obtained with apparent molecular weights of 45–50, 23 and 15 kD. Similar results were recently obtained by immunoprecipitation, and moreover eosinophil FcεRII was compared with CD23. Whereas BB10 precipitated three polypeptides of apparent M_r 45–50, 20–25 and 15 kD on eosinophils and on a B cell line (WIL-2WT), a mAb anti CD23 (mAb135 kindly provided by Dr G. Delespesse, University of Montreal, Canada) bound to a major 45–50 kD component both on eosinophils and on WIL-2WT cells. This study together with previous results confirms the existence of a common structure between FcεRII present on eosinophils, platelets, macrophages and B-lymphocytes [9]. On occasion, it has been argued that the low affinity of this second receptor could lessen its real biological significance in IgE-dependent reactions. In fact, the affinity observed for monomeric IgE is comparable with or even higher than the affinity generally reported for the IgG receptors. On the other hand, the increased extrinsic affinity of FcεRII for IgE dimers or complexes gives this class of receptors a particular significance in all situations where IgE complexes are produced, such as parasitic infections and allergic diseases [reviewed in 9]. In this respect, our demonstration of surface-bound IgE to rat and human eosinophils indicates that in spite of the low affinity of FcεRII for monomeric IgE *in vitro,* IgE immunoglobulins are able to bind to eosinophil FcεRII *in vivo.*

Receptors for IgA

Whereas receptors for IgA have been detected on various leucocyte populations, their presence has not been reported on normal human eosinophils. The recent demonstration of surface IgE and IgA on intestinal eosinophils from parasite infected mice [13] or on blood eosinophils from patients with filariasis [14] suggested the existence of receptors for IgA on activated eosinophils. The binding of monomeric IgA to purified human eosinophils (> 95% purity) was evaluated by flow cytofluorometry analysis after staining with fluorescein-labelled antihuman IgA. Between 5 and 60% of eosinophils were able to bind IgA. Moreover, the proportion of surface IgA bearing eosinophils increased in the case of allergic patients [15]. These results very interestingly showed similarities between the percentages of eosinophils able to bind IgE and IgA. The association between the two receptors at the level of individual cells is currently under investigation.

Receptors for IgM

The existence of a receptor for IgM on human eosinophils is still debated, and its detection seems dependent upon precise technical parameters [3,16].

Release of mediators upon Ig-dependent activation

IgG-dependent activation

The functional aspects of IgG receptors have been first evidenced in ADCC mechanisms. The appropriate triggering of human eosinophils by IgG antibodies coated to parasite targets induced the lysis, involving cationic proteins such as MBP or ECP, as well as oxidative metabolism [reviewed in 1]. This IgG-mediated ADCC mechanism is strongly enhanced by a variety of factors such as eosinophil activating factor (EAF), granulocyte macrophage-colony stimulating factor (GM-CSF), PAF-acether, tumour necrosis factor (TNF) or endothelial cell supernatants [reviewed in 9]. However, very few studies have concerned their direct effects on the IgG receptor itself. The triggering of eosinophil IgG receptors by human IgG coated on Sepharose beads, induces the release of LTC_4 and higher amounts are generated by hypodense eosinophils [17]. However, increased levels of LTC_4 are obtained when normodense eosinophils are activated by FMLP or EAF [17]. Similar results were obtained with IgG antibodies directed against *Aspergillus fumigatus* in the presence of the specific antigen. The production of H_2O_2 in response to IgG-dependent stimulation has also been reported [18]. Eosinophils release twice as much H_2O_2 as do neutrophils upon interaction with IgG1-, IgG2- or IgG3-coated Sepharose beads, but this difference becomes fivefold with IgG4-coated Sepharose [18]. This favours the view of distinct functional interactions between eosinophil IgG receptors and the IgG subclasses.

IgE-dependent activation

The demonstration of surface IgE on eosinophils from patients with increased IgE levels and particularly on lung eosinophils confirmed the biological relevance of the interaction between eosinophils and IgE antibodies [5]. In order to investigate the role of these cytophilic IgE in eosinophil function and to evaluate their specificity, further experiments measuring the release of various mediators were then performed.

Eosinophil peroxidase was detected in the supernatants of eosinophils from hypereosinophilic patients after incubation either with the specific antigen or with anti-IgE antibodies. This was obtained not only in the case of patients with filarial infections [19] but more recently confirmed in the case of allergic patients [14]. Only allergens related to the patient's allergy and giving positivity in the skin tests induced extracellular release of EPO. However no release of EPO was obtained when the same allergens were added to eosinophils from non-allergic patients. Not only EPO but also MBP was released after addition of anti-IgE antibodies [14]. These results suggest that cell-bound IgE with very restricted antibody specificity could play a role in the activation of hypodense eosinophils in inducing the release of granule proteins with potent cytolytic functions.

Selectivity of mediator release

Eosinophil peroxidase and MBP were released after addition of anti-IgE but not anti-IgG antibodies. In contrast, ECP measured by a radioimmunoassay using monoclonal antibodies (EG1, kindly performed by Dr P.C. Tai, London) was only detected after addition of anti-IgG antibodies. These results showing no correlation between EPO and ECP release suggested a variability in the response of eosinophils to different stimuli (IgE versus IgG). Similar results have been recently reported concerning a differential release of EPO and ECP in response to activation by opsonized zymosan [20].

They were more recently confirmed by studies on a factor named HRF (histamine releasing factor) able to induce histamine release after addition to IgE-bearing basophils [21]. When surface IgE bearing eosinophils were incubated with partly purified HRF factor, EPO was detected in the supernatants but not ECP, similarly to the IgE-dependent activation. These results show that the release of eosinophil mediators can be induced not only by antigens or anti-IgE but also by soluble factors such as HRF. Histamine releasing factor, which is present in nasal lavage fluids and blister fluids during the late cutaneous reaction, has a molecular weight of 15–30 kD, and can be considered in some aspects as an 'IgE binding factor'. It is produced *in vitro* by lung macrophages and platelets, both cell populations bearing in common the second receptor for IgE (FcεRII). However no similar studies have been related with the production of such IgE binding factors by eosinophils. In preliminary experiments we have recently shown that FcεR+ hypodense eosinophils are able to release soluble factors of a molecular weight comparable with the previously described IgE binding factors, and able to bind IgE [9].

Finally, the production of a newly formed mediator such as PAF-acether in response to IgE-dependent triggering, but not to IgG-dependent stimulation of hypodense eosinophils confirm the selectivity in the mediators produced by eosinophils according to the stimulus of activation [22]. These findings have to be considered in relation to human eosinophil heterogeneity. Indeed it has been recently shown that lung eosinophils produced 1000-fold more PAF-acether in response to anti-IgE antibodies than corresponding blood eosinophils from the same patients [23]. Moreover normodense eosinophils seemed to produce significant although limited amounts of PAF, in response to IgG triggering and not to IgE triggering [24].

IgA-dependent activation

The existence of surface IgA bound to eosinophils from allergic or parasite-infected patients led us to investigate the IgA-dependent release of mediators. Eosinophil peroxidase was evaluated after addition of anti-IgA antibodies to highly purified eosinophils. A significant release of EPO (between 2.5 and 6 times more than in controls) were obtained after addition of anti-IgA. These results suggested that similarly to IgE, surface IgA could participate in eosinophil activation, by inducing the release of mediators [15]. Further experiments are in progress to determine the respective role of IgA and IgE receptors in the effector function of eosinophils.

The majority of studies dealing with eosinophil functions have been performed in parasitic infections or in allergic diseases. In addition to previous reports suggesting the role of eosinophils in such situations (increased numbers of eosinophils in the biological fluids or detection of specific eosinophil mediators in the lavage or on tissue sections), our results show that eosinophils, through their surface immunoglobulins are able to interact with antigens, and to release their various mediators. Among the various immunoglobulin isotypes, surface IgE and IgA seem particularly involved in mediator release and these findings may have *in vivo* implications in the context of tissue reactions, specially in the lungs and in the intestine.

Electron microscopy studies

Taken all together, these results suggesting a differential release of eosinophil granule mediators in response to a given stimulus of activation, seem incompatible with the hypothesis of exocytosis of the whole granules. Recent studies using electron microscopy and immunogold staining rather suggest a release process of the individual components from the granules through the cytoplasm [25]. Tissue eosinophils from a patient suffering from eosinophilic gastroenteritis, with a story of milk allergy, were analysed by immunogold staining with the appropriate specific antibodies directed against MBP, EPO (kindly donated by Dr Venge, Uppsala, Sweden), or ECP (EG2, kindly provided by Dr Tai in London). In ulcerated areas, MBP was virtually absent from the crystalloid, but detected in the matrix and out of the granules, whereas EPO and ECP were still present in the matrix of the granules [25]. These findings bring morphologic evidence consistent with the hypothesis of a selective release of granule constituents from activated eosinophils. They suggest that the inversion of the electron density of the granule crystalloid, reported by several authors is due to a loss of MBP. The precise mechanisms for the induction of eosinophil degranulation are unknown and further *in vitro* studies are now undertaken to follow the kinetics of eosinophil degranulation in response to given stimuli.

Therapeutic implications

The participation of eosinophils in the cellular network during allergy and more generally inflammatory reactions led to consider new therapeutical approaches in order to decrease or abolish the deleterious effects of eosinophils and their mediators. The major steps of eosinophil activation might represent the targets of such drugs: the attraction of eosinophils by chemotactic factors, the stage of activation by various stimuli, and the release of mediators. Very recently, the strong inhibitory effect of a new antihistamine, antiallergic drug (cetirizine), on eosinophil chemotaxis induced by PAF or by FMLP has been reported [26]. Similarly, the specific ginkgolide-derived PAF antagonist, BN52021, strongly inhibited the PAF-induced chemotaxis (27]. Interestingly these two drugs have limited effects on neutrophils. It could also be envisaged to selectively inhibit the activation signal due to IgE triggering. Indeed, disodium cromoglycate (DSCG) was shown to inhibit the chemiluminescence reaction induced by addition of anti-IgE but not by anti-IgG or phorbol esters, to eosinophils from asthmatic patients. It is noteworthy to point out that DSCG has similar effects on macrophages and platelets [28], whereas the inhibition of IgE-dependent release of mediators from human lung mast-cells is surprisingly weak [reviewed in 29]. However, DSCG totally inhibited the FMLP-induced eosinophil activation, as evaluated by complement and IgG rosettes or complement-dependent cytotoxicity [29]. Finally, the potent inhibition of eosinophil-mediated IgE-dependent cytotoxicity, but at a lesser extent of IgG-mediated cytotoxicity by PAF-antagonists [22], tend to support our working hypothesis of selectivity of mediator release.

Corticosteroids are the most effective drugs for the treatment of chronic asthma. However hypereosinophilic patients do not always respond favourably to corticosteroid therapy, especially patients with malignant hypereosinophilic syndrome (HES). In this respect, we have recently shown that eosinophils from corticoresistant patients were lacking the receptor for corticosteroids, both by radiolabelled hormone binding assay or by the use of a specific anti-receptor monoclonal antibody [30]. These data provide evidence that the presence of corticosteroid receptors is a prerequisite for corticosteroid activity and may provide valuable information on corticosteroid sensitivity.

Conclusion

In conclusion, these studies appear to have opened a new cellular pathway in the mechanisms of hypersensitivity reactions. The demonstration of receptors for IgE and now for IgA on eosinophils has certainly broadened our current view on the cellular mechanisms of allergic reactions. The further demonstration that the activation of these receptors is associated with the selectivity and the dynamics of pharmacological mediator release might have significant implication in our understanding of the physiopathology of allergic and inflammatory reactions but also in the definition of novel therapeutic strategies.

References

1 Gleich GJ, Adolphson CR. The eosinophilic leukocyte. *Adv. Immunol.* 1986;**39**:177–253.

2 Butterworth AE, Remold HG, Houba V, David JR, Franks D, David PH, Sturrock RF. Antibody dependent eosinophil mediated damage to ^{51}Cr labeled schistosomula of *S. mansoni*: mediation by IgG and inhibition by antigen-antibody complexes. *J. Immunol.* 1977;**118**:2230–2236.

3 Walsh GM, Kay AB. Binding of immunoglobulin classes and subclasses to human neutrophils and eosinophils. *Clin. Exp. Immunol.* 1986;**63**:466–472.

4 Khalife J, Capron M, Grzych JM, Bazin H, Capron A. Fc receptors on rat eosinophils: isotype-dependent cell activation. *J. Immunol.* 1985;**135**:2780–2784.

5 Capron M, Kusnierz JP, Prin L, Spiegelberg HL, Ovlaque G, Gosset P, Tonnel AB, Capron A. Cytophilic IgE on human blood and tissue eosinophils: detection by flow microfluorometry. *J. Immunol.* 1985;**134**:3013–3018.

6 Kulczycki, A. Jr. Human neutrophils and eosinophils have structurally distinct Fc receptors. *J. Immunol.* 1984;**133**:849–854.

7 Capron M, Capron A, Goetzl EJ, Austen KF. Tetrapeptides of the eosinophil chemotactic factor of anaphylaxis (ECF-A) enhance eosinophil Fc receptor. *Nature* 1981;**289**:71–73.

8 Kay AB, Walsh GM. Chemotactic factor-induced enhancement of the binding of human immunoglobulin classes and subclasses to neutrophils and eosinophils. *Clin. Exp. Immunol.* 1984;**57**:729–734.

9 Capron M, Grangette C, Torpier G, Capron A. The second receptor for IgE in eosinophil effector function. *Chemical Immunology* 1989;**47**:128–178.

10 Capron M, Jouault T, Prin L, Joseph M, Ameisen JC, Butterworth AE, Papin JP, Kusnierz JP, Capron A. Functional study of a monoclonal antibody to IgE Fc receptor (FcεRII) of eosinophils, platelets and macrophages. *J. Exp. Med.* 1986;**164**:72–89.

11 Capron M, Kazatchkine MD, Fischer E, Joseph M, Butterworth AE, Kusnierz JP, Prin L, Papin JP, Capron A. Functional role of the α-chain of complement receptor type 3 in human eosinophil-dependent antibody-mediated cytotoxicity against schistosomes. *J. Immunol.* 1987;**139**:2059–2065.

12 Jouault T, Capron M, Balloul JM, Ameisen JC, Capron A. Quantitative and qualitative analysis of the Fc receptor for IgE (FcεRII) on human eosinophils. *Eur. J. Immunol.* 1988;**18**:237–241.

13 Van der Vorst E, Dhont H, Cesbron JY, Capron M, Dessaint JP, Capron A. The influence of an *Hymenolepis diminuta* infection on the IgE and IgA bound to mouse intestinal eosinophils. *Int. Arch. Allergy Appl. Immunol.* 1988;**87,3**;281–285.

14 Capron M, Leprevost C, Prin L, Tomassini M, Torpier G, MacDonald S, Capron A. Immunoglobulin-mediated activation of eosinophils. In *Eosinophils in Asthma* (Eds Morley J, Colditz I), Academic Press, London, 1989, pp. 49–60.

15 Capron M, Tomassini M, Van der Vorst E, Kusnierz JP, Papin JP, Capron A. Existence et fonctions d'un récepteur pour l'IgA sur les éosinophiles humains. *CR Acad. Sci.* 1988;**307** (série III):397–402.

16 De Simone C, Donelli G, Meli D, Molinari A, Rosati F, Sorice F. Human peripheral eosinophils with receptors for IgM: demonstration and ultrastructural morphology. *Immunobiology* 1982;**162**:116–127.

17 Wardlaw AJ, Kay AB. The role of the eosinophil in pathogenesis of asthma. *Allergy* 1987;**42**:321–335.

18 Yazdanbaksh M, Eckmann CM, Roos D. Characterization of the interaction of human eosinophils and neutrophils with opsonized particles. *J. Immunol.* 1985;**135**:1378–1384.

19 Khalife J, Capron M, Cesbron JY, Tai PC, Taelman H, Prin L, Capron A. Role of specific IgE antibodies in peroxidase (EPO) release from human eosinophils *J. Immunol.* 1986;**137**:1659–1664.

20 Venge P. Eosinophil biochemistry and killing mechanisms. In: *Eosinophils in Asthma* (Eds Morley J, Colditz I), Academic Press, London, 1989, pp. 49–60.

21 Liu MC, Proud D, Lichtenstein LM, MacGlashan DW Jr, Schleimer RP, Adkinson NF Jr, Kagey-Sobotka A, Schulman ES, Plaut M. Human lung macrophage-derived histamine-releasing activity is due to IgE dependent factors. *J. Immunol.* 1986;**136**:2588–2595.

22 Capron M, Benveniste J, Braquet P, Capron A. Role of PAF-acether in IgE-dependent activation of eosinophils. In: *New Trends in Lipid Mediators Research* Vol. 2 (Ed. Braquet J), Karger, Basel;1988: pp. 10–17.

23 Bruynzeel PLB, Verhagen J. Lipid metabolism by eosinophils. In *Eosinophils in Asthma* (Eds Morley J, Colditz I), Academic Press, London, 1989, pp. 49–60.

24 Kay AB, Frew AJ, Moqbel R, Walsh GM, Kurihara K, Cromwell O, Champion A, Hartnell A, Wardlaw AJ. The activated eosinophil in allergy and asthma. In *Biochemistry of the Acute Allergic Reactions,* Vth International Symposium, (Eds Tauber AI, Wintroub BU, Simon AS), Alan R Liss Inc, New York, 1989, pp. 183–197.

25 Torpier G., Colombel JF, Mathieu-Chandelier C, Capron M, Dessaint JP, Cortot A, Paris JC, Capron. A Eosinophilic gastroenteritis: Ultrastructural evidence for a selective release of eosinophil major basic protein. *Clin. Exp. Immunol.* 1988;**74,3**:404–408.

26 Leprevost C, Capron M, De Vos C, Tomassini M, Capron A. Inhibition of eosinophil chemotaxis by a new antiallergic compound (cetirizine). *Int. Arch. Allergy Appl. Immunol.* 1988;**87**:9–13.

27 Kurihara K, Wardlaw AJ, Moqbel R, Kay AB. Inhibition of PAF-induced chemotaxis and PAF-binding to human eosinophils and neutrophils by the specific ginkgolide-derived PAF antagonist, BN52021. *J. Allergy Clin. Immunol.* 1989;**83,1**:83–90.

28 Tsicopoulos A, Lassalle P, Joseph M, Tonnel AB, Thorel T, Dessaint JP, Capron A. Effect of disodium cromoglycate on inflammatory cells bearing the FcεRII. *Int. J. Immunopharmacol.* 1988;**10**:227–236.

29 Kay AB, Walsh GM, Moqbel R, MacDonald AJ, Nagakura T, Carroll MP, Richerson HB. Disodium cromoglycate inhibits activation of human inflammatory cells *in vitro*. *J. Allergy. Clin. Immunol.* 1987;**80**:1–8.

30 Prin L, Lefebvre P, Gruart V, Capron M, Formstecher D, Loiseau S, Capron A. Heterogeneity of human eosinophil glucocorticoid receptor expression in hypereosinophilic patients: absence of receptor correlates with resistance to corticotherapy. *Clin. Exp. Immunol.* 1989;**78**:383–389.

3 · Interleukin-5: molecular biology and function

Elaine J. Clutterbuck and C.J. Sanderson

Introduction

The possibility that the control of eosinophilia is mediated by a lymphokine was initially suggested by the T-cell dependence of eosinophilia induced by parasites in rats [1] and by observations that supernatants of activated spleen cells can induce eosinophil colony formation [2]. For these reasons we sought to identify the activity produced by mouse T-cells, which was stimulating eosinophil production *in vitro*. A stable T-cell hybrid (NIMP-TH1) was produced from spleen cells of mice undergoing parasite-induced eosinophilia. On stimulation with phorbol myristate acetate this hybrid released a soluble activity, which selectively stimulated eosinophil production from murine bone marrow [3], and was therefore termed eosinophil differentiation factor (EDF). Coordinate analysis of the production of lymphokines by primary alloreactive T-cell clones revealed a highly significant correlation between eosinophil differentiation activity and B-cell growth factor II (BCGFII) activity [4]. These two activities copurified through a series of protein separation techniques [5], and led to its designation as interleukin-5 (IL-5).

Although there are several reports of native human eosinophil colony stimulating factors (CSFs) and BCGFs of similar high molecular weight to murine IL-5 [6,7], no native human equivalent of murine IL-5 has been characterized. The cloning of the murine factor however led to the cloning and expression of the analogous human factor.

Characterization of IL-5

EDF from NIMP-TH1 appeared after gel filtration as a heterogeneous band with a peak at M_r 46 000 [8]. The activity was destroyed by trypsin, and bound to immobilized lentil lectin, suggesting it was a glycoprotein. When the cells were grown in the presence of tunicamycin, which blocks *N*-linked glycosylation, the activity eluted with a M_r 30 000 indicating a maximum size for the protein, and suggesting that the carbohydrate was not essential for biological activity.

A cDNA expression library was produced from NIMP-TH1 mRNA and screened by expression in COS cells. A cDNA clone was identified by assaying the COS cell supernatant for EDF activity [9]. The cDNA contained a single open reading frame coding for a polypeptide of 133 amino acids, identical to the sequence reported for TRF/BCGFII [10]. The expression product strongly stimulated both the eosinophil lineage and showed BCGFII activity, thus confirming our original report that EDF and BCGFII were properties of a single molecule [5].

Structure of the IL-5 gene

The mouse IL-5 cDNA coding region fragment was used as a probe for Southern blotting and isolation of the mouse and human genes from genomic lambda libraries. The sequence of the human and murine genes showed that the relative positions of the introns in the coding sequence were identical [9,11]. The introns all begin with GT and end in AG. Areas of high homology were identified in all the introns, although in the mouse the first two introns were considerably larger than in the human gene. Mouse IL-5 mRNA is much larger than its human counterpart because of 738 additional untranslated bases 3′ of the termination codon. Apart from this the exons are highly conserved.

There is no significant homology between the mouse IL-5 gene sequence and other genes encoding haemopoietic growth factors, except for a region upstream of the TATA boxes. This region is present in both mouse and human IL-5 and granulocyte macrophage colony-stimulating factor (GM-CSF) genes, human GC-SF and murine IL-4 genes [12]. This preserved 10-base sequence may represent a regulatory element for this group of lymphokines active in haemopoiesis.

The human IL-5 gene is located at chromosome 5q31 and is deleted in patients with the 5q- syndrome [13]. The genes for IL-3 and GM-CSF have also been located to this region of chromosome 5 [12,14], and the murine IL-4 gene lies near the analogous area on chromosome 11 [15]. The genes encoding all these four factors share an overall structural similarity with similar exon sizes. These similarities within the genes and their clustering on one chromosome raise interesting possibilities for their evolution and regulation.

Structure of the IL-5 protein

The IL-5 genes encode precursors of 133 amino acids in the mouse and 134 in man. Amino acids 1–20 in the mouse serve as a signal sequence for the gene, leaving a maximum polypeptide length of 113 amino acids with an M_r of about 12 000 [16,17]. The predicted site of cleavage of the human signal peptide is after amino acid 19, to give a processed protein of 115 amino acids (M_r is about 13 000) [12]. As expected for a secreted protein a long hydrophobic stretch preceded by a basic residue is present at the N terminus. As discussed above the native mouse protein appears to be of approximately M_r 30 000 in the non-glycosylated form, and so is likely to be a dimer. There are three potential *N*-glycosylation sites in the mouse IL-5, the first and last of which are conserved in the human protein. Two cysteine residues are present in each mature protein at corresponding positions. There is a high amino acid sequence identity between mouse and human IL-5 (67%). This contrasts with only 29% between mouse and human IL-3 and 52% between mouse and human GM-CSF.

Biological activity of IL-5

As a murine eosinophil differentiation factor

Recombinant murine IL-5 (rmIL-5) exactly mimics the activity of the native molecule. IL-5 is a lineage specific growth and differentiation factor for eosinophils [8,9].

In semi-solid agar cultures mIL-5 selectively stimulates the production of a few eosinophil colonies from murine fetal liver cells [18] and bone marrow from parasitized mice [9]. Liquid murine bone marrow cultures have a higher sensitivity for detecting mIL-5 than semi-solid colony assays. Marrow from mice infected with *Mesocestoides corti* produced at least 10-fold the number of eosinophils than normal bone marrow. Eosinophil production was transient (8–9 weeks) but at peak production the cultures from infected mice contained about 80–90% eosinophils [8]. Under both light and electron microscope these were typical eosinophils, although the nuclear structure indicated that only a minority were fully mature.

To investigate the biological role of IL-5 in the production of eosinophilia *in vivo,* assays were carried out at different times after infection with *M. corti.* The development of eosinophilia in these infected mice was preceded by detectable levels of mIL-5 in the serum. No mIL-3 could be detected in serum samples at any stage of the infection [19]. This detection of IL-5 in serum suggests a biological role for this factor in the development of eosinophilia.

As a human eosinophil differentiation factor

mIL-5 shows cross-species reactivity for the eosinophil lineage, stimulating the production of eosinophils from normal human bone marrow, with no effect on other cell types [18,20]. In contrast to the action of mIL-5 on normal murine bone marrow, semi-solid culture of normal human bone marrow is as sensitive as liquid culture in the detection of mIL-5 [20]. Clone transfer experiments and the linear relationship between the number of bone marrow cells plated and colonies produced confirmed that the action of mIL-5 was directly on eosinophil progenitor cells, not through an intermediary action on accessory cells [18].

The time-course of human eosinophil production by mIL-5 and rhIL-5, as well as rhIL-3 and rhGM-CSF, was similar. Significant numbers of eosinophils develop in liquid culture of normal human bone marrow after 7–14 days, reaching a peak after 3–4 weeks, when eosinophils were the predominant cell type [21].

The ability to culture eosinophils *in vitro* under controlled conditions by these cytokines has facilitated the study of their morphological maturation. Until the third week most of the eosinophils were typical myelocytes. Thereafter they developed into metamyelocytes until mature eosinophils developed after about 6–7 weeks. All cell types had characteristic light- and electron-microscopic features.

Although our studies with murine cultures have not been so detailed, the persistence in culture of eosinophils with 'doughnut' nuclei suggest that final maturation may be delayed in that system as well. This appears to contrast with the rapid appearance of mature eosinophils *in vivo*. Eosinophilia appears 1–2 weeks after ingestion of food infected with *Trichinella spiralis* and peaks at the end of the third week [22]. Herion [23] suggested a mean marrow transit time of 9 days and a post-mitotic transit time of 2½ days in normal subjects and patients with eosinophilia. While this difference is not understood, margination from tissue pools also contributes to blood eosinophilia *in vivo,* and so the kinetics are not directly comparable.

It has been postulated from observations of marrow aspirates [24,25] that dense 'primary' eosinophil granules in myelocytes result from condensation of the flocculent contents of the membrane-lined vacuoles present in promyelocytes. 'Primary' granules were then thought to develop into the smaller 'secondary' granules usually seen in circulating mature eosinophils, which have crystalloid cores. We have followed the differentiation of granules and confirm that primary granules first appear as vacuoles containing flocculent material. Like Scott and Horn [25], dense material resembling granule matrix in the Golgi lamellae were not seen. Although the vacuoles occasionally resembled adjacent areas of dilated ER, the origin of these granules remains unclear.

The granules present in the mature cells were similar in size to mature secondary granules (0.45 ± 0.17 μm) [26], but none of the cytokines produced granules with classical crystalline cores. A few had lamellae parallel to the granule surface which might be an early stage of crystallization [27]. The crystalloid core of mature granules contains major basic protein (MBP) [28], which is present in the granules of eosinophil myelocytes induced *in vitro* by both rhIL-5 and rhIL-3 [29]. As these eosinophils exhibit normal functional activity [20], it is possible that this 'abnormal' appearance of the MBP may be a culture artefact rather than truncated differentiation.

As an eosinophil-activating factor

Both mIL-5 and rhIL-5 increased the capacity of normal human peripheral blood eosinophils to kill antibody-coated tumour cells, phagocytose serum-opsonized yeast cells, and to produce superoxide anion [18,30]. This activation was accompanied by morphological changes such that they became irregular in shape, the membrane ruffled and the granules concentrated on one end (polarization) [30]. The *in vitro* survival of human eosinophils, but not neutrophils was prolonged by mIL-5 [31]. Similar activation by mIL-5 of eosinophils from parasitized mice have also been shown [32,33], and mIL-5 may have weak chemotactic properties [33].

Although not fully morphologically mature (see above), the eosinophils produced *in vitro* by IL-5 had reached functional maturity. Murine eosinophils were cytotoxic towards antibody-coated erythrocytes, and killed schistosomula of *Schistosoma mansoni* in the presence of antibody and complement [8,34]. Human eosinophils produced *in vitro* by either mIL-5 or rhIL-5 were also cytotoxic to antibody-coated tumour cells [20, and unpublished work]. Interestingly, functional activity was present to the same degree in both cultured immature eosinophil myelocytes and mature cells, with little enhancement of cytotoxicity being inducible by the presence of IL-5 in the assay. This suggests that eosinophil activation is not the final step in differentiation, but may be a separate pathway [20].

mIL-5 is a murine B-cell growth factor

mIL-5 acts as a BCGFII stimulating the proliferation of B-cells co-stimulated with dextran sulphate [35], naturally occurring large B-cells (which have presumably been preactivated *in vivo*), and the mouse B-cell lymphoma BCL_1 [36]. In addition it is a differentiating factor stimulating the production of IgM and IgG from these cells [36].

mIL-5 also induces a three- to sixfold increase in IgA production by LPS-stimulated splenic B-cells, together with a less than twofold increase in other isotypes [37–40]. mIL-4 potentiates the IgA-enhancing activity of mIL-5 [37,38]. It is not clear whether mIL-5 acts on precommitted B-cells as a class switch factor for IgA or as a maturation factor for surface IgA positive ($sIgA^+$) cells, promoting their proliferation or inducing terminal differentiation into IgA secreting cells. Several studies report that mIL-5 does not act on sIgA negative splenic or Peyers patch B-cells but stimulates $sIgA^+$ cells to differentiate to high rate IgA synthesis [39,41,42].

Failure to detect activity of rhIL-5 on human B-cells

The activity of mIL-5 as a BCGFII suggested that the human B-cell growth factors of similar high molecular weight (BCGF-H) [6,7] may have represented native forms of human IL-5. rhIL-5 was therefore tested in a panel of standard B-cell assays used to identify BCGFs in man. Purified rhIL-5 of high EDF activity was used in case other confounding activities existed in COS cell supernatants. This material did not have inhibitory activity in a B-cell assay using commercially available low molecular weight BCGF (BCGF-L) [43].

Although rhIL-5 was active on the mouse BCL_1 cell line, no detectable activity on any of the panel of assays was demonstrable [44]. These included: proliferation assays with tonsillar or splenic B-cells in the presence of the stimulators anti-μ, PMA, SAC or a mixture of PDB and Ionomycin; proliferation of BCGF responsive cell lines; IgM or IgG production by tonsillar B-cells stimulated by SAC or PMA, the CESS cell line; and finally its ability to replace T-cells in specific antibody responses, measuring the production of IgM, IgG and IgA. All the B-cell preparations were of > 95% purity.

This contrasts with other reports that rhIL-5 induces human B-cell differentiation [40,45]. Both used unpurified material, and the small increases demonstrated were not statistically evaluated. The B-cell preparation used by Yokota *et al.* [40] contained 50% T-cells and 5% monocytes. Recent work has demonstrated that rhIL-5 did not induce significant IgA production by highly purified human splenic B-cells. Moreover the IgA inducing effects of rhIL-5 demonstrable in enriched B-cell populations were probably indirectly mediated via T-cells, which could be replaced by IL-2.

rhIL-5 does not therefore have activity analogous to murine BCGFII or TRF, and the BCGF-H do not represent native forms of IL-5. There is no good evidence that rhIL-5 acts directly on B-cells, and all the reported activities appear to be dependent on the presence of accessory cells.

The role of IL-5 in the regulation of eosinophil haemopoiesis

Neutrophil growth factors can support long-term production of neutrophils apparently due to the maintenance of stem cell proliferation and the continued production of neutrophil precursors [46]. In both murine and human cultures the production of eosinophils was relatively transient (see above). It appears therefore that IL-5 may not be stimulating a similar production of eosinophil precursors *in vitro,* but is active only on precursor cells pre-committed to the eosinophil lineage. It is presumed that the enhanced eosinophil production induced by IL-5 from parasitized bone marrow is due to the presence of more committed precursors.

The relative insensitivity of murine colony assays hindered the study of the regulation of murine precursor cells until the development of a method for enriching primitive stem cells. Pretreatment of mice with 5-fluorouracil (5-FU) depletes their marrow and spleens of mature cells and *in vitro* colony-forming units (CFU). The cells remaining are enriched for an early stem cell population which generates very large colonies ($> 5\times10^4$ cells) in semi-solid agar cultures. mIL-5 did not induce eosinophil colony formation from such preparations [32,47]. mIL-3 supported the formation of multilineage colonies, 44% of which contained eosinophils [32]. Secondary semi-solid culture of mIL-3-induced blast cells with mIL-5 resulted in the formation of some IL-5-responsive eosinophil colonies [47]. mIL-5 in contrast to IL-3 therefore appeared not to act on primitive murine cells. The role of IL-5 was to promote terminal differentiation and proliferation of cells already committed to the eosinophil lineage.

Semi-solid cultures of unfractionated normal human bone marrow are sufficiently sensitive to study the role of rhIL-5 in human haemopoiesis. The number of eosinophil clusters (groups of more than four cells) present in semi-solid cultures gives an estimation of the numbers of progenitors. Only those progenitors stimulated to form clusters of more than 40 cells are designated CFU.

A small number of eosinophil clusters are present in semi-solid cultures grown in the absence of an external source of CSF. This is presumably due to factors present in the fetal calf serum or produced spontaneously by accessory cells. rhIL-3 or rhGM-CSF, but not rhIL-5, increased the number of eosinophil clusters [21]. Using a two-step assay system, liquid preculture with rhIL-3 or rhGM-CSF but not rhIL-5, rhIL-1 or rhIL-6 enhances the production of eosinophil colonies responsive to either rhIL-5, rhIL-3 or rhGM-CSF in secondary semi-solid cultures [48]. Taken together these data support the hypothesis that rhIL-5 (unlike rhIL-3 or rhGM-CSF) is unable to generate eosinophil precursors from uncommitted human stem cells. It should be stressed that both rhIL-3 and rhGM-CSF also enhanced the production and subsequent proliferation of both neutrophil and macrophage precursors.

The relative activities of rhIL-5, rhIL-3 and rhGM-CSF on the regulation of human eosinophil haemopoiesis *in vitro* is complex. IL-5 is the only cytokine selective for the eosinophil lineage. In colony cultures optimal doses of either rhIL-3 or rhGM-CSF stimulate more eosinophil colony production than rhIL-5. Co-culturing rhIL-5 with either rhIL-3 or rhGM-CSF increased the number of eosinophil colonies, but only to the sum of colony numbers induced by the individual factors alone [21]. The action of rhIL-5 was therefore additive to, but not synergistic with the other cytokines. These data suggest that rhIL-5 may stimulate a smaller and possibly different pool of eosinophil progenitors from rhIL-3 or rhGM-CSF. Similar results were found in liquid cultures experiments.

In contrast, rhIL-5 stimulates the production of more eosinophils in liquid cultures than either rhIL-3 or rhGM-CSF [21]. These contrasting data from the two different culture systems appear to indicate that while rhIL-5 may act on fewer precursors than rhIL-3 or rhGM-CSF, it might cause more proliferative steps and so produce more eosinophils.

Conclusion

The biological role of IL-5 as a B-cell growth factor is unclear. In mice this activity is readily detectable *in vitro*. Although IgE antibody is associated with eosinophilia, current evidence indicates that IL-4 rather than IL-5 is active in IgE induction, although rhIL-5 enhances the T- and monocyte-dependent IgE production by rhIL-4 from human B-cells [49].

The role of cytokines in the production of eosinophilia is complex. If rhIL-3 or rhGM-CSF play a significant role in the production of eosinophil precursors, the selective eosinophilia observed *in vivo* (without a concomitant increase in neutrophils and macrophages) requires other regulatory mechanisms. This role could be fulfilled by rhIL-5 which is selective for the eosinophil lineage even though it seems unable to generate its own precursors. Some support for a biological role for IL-5 in the induction of eosinophilia comes from its appearance in the serum of mice during eosinophilia induced by a parasitic infection; however as yet there is no reported evidence for a role in man.

References

1 Basten A, Beeson PB. Mechanism of eosinophilia. II Role of the lymphocyte. *J. Exp. Med.* 1970;**131**:1288.

2 Metcalf D, Parker JW, Chester HM, Kincade, PW. Formation of eosinophilic-like granulocytic colonies by mouse bone marrow cells *in vitro*. *J. Cell. Physiol.* 1974;**84**:275.

3 Warren DJ, Sanderson, CJ. Production of a T cell hybrid producing a lymphokine stimulating eosinophil differentiation. *Immunology* 1985;**54**:615.

4 Sanderson CJ, Strath M, Warren DJ, O'Garra A, Kirkwood TBL. The production of lymphokines by primary alloreactive T cell clones. A co-ordinate analysis of 233 clones in seven lymphokine assays. *Immunology* 1985;**56**:575.

5 Sanderson CJ, O'Garra A, Warren DJ, Klaus GGB. Eosinophil differentiation factor also has B cell growth factor activity. Proposed name interleukin 4. *Proc. Natl. Acad. Sci. USA* 1986;**83**:437.

6 Yoshizaki K, Nakagawa T, Fukunaga K, Tseng LT, Yamamura Y, Kishimoto T. Isolation and characterisation of B cell differentiation factor (BCDF) secreted from a human lymphoblastoid cell line. *J. Immunol.* 1984;**132**:2948.

7 Ambrus JL, Jurgensen CH, Brown EJ, Fauci AS. Purification to homogeneity of a high molecular weight human B cell growth factor; demonstration of specific binding to activated B cells; and development of a monoclonal antibody to the factor *J. Exp. Med.* 1985;**162**:1319.

8 Sanderson CJ, Warren DJ, Strath M. Identification of a lymphokine that stimulates eosinophil differentiation *in vitro*. Its relationship to IL3, and functional properties of eosinophils produced in cultures. *J. Exp. Med.* 1985;**162**:60.

9 Campbell HD, Sanderson CJ, Wang Y, Hort Y, Martinson ME, Tucker WQJ, Stellwagen A, Strath M, Young IG. Isolation, structure and expression of cDNA and genomic clones for murine eosinophil differentiation factor. Comparison with other eosinophilopoietic lymphokines and identity with interleukin-5. *Eur. J. Biochem.* 1988;**174**:345.

10 Kinashi T, Harada N, Severinson E, Tanabe T, Sideras P, Konishi M, Azuma C, Tominaga A, Bergstedt-Lindqvist S, Takahashi M, Matsuda F, Yaoita Y, Takatsu K, Honjo T. Cloning of a complementary DNA encoding T-cell replacing factor and identity with B-cell growth factor II. *Nature* 1986;**324**:70.

11 Campbell HD, Tucker WQJ, Hort Y, Martinson ME, Mayo G, Clutterbuck EJ, Sanderson CJ, Young IG. Molecular cloning, nucleotide sequence, and expression of the gene encoding human eosinophil differentiation factor (interleukin-5). *Proc. Natl. Acad. Sci. USA* 1987;**84**:6629.

12 Sanderson CJ, Campbell HD, Young IG. Molecular and cellular biology of eosinophil differentiation factor (Interleukin-5) and its effects on human and mouse B cells. *Immunol. Rev.* 1988;**102**:29.

13 Sutherland GR, Baker E, Callen DF, Campbell HD, Young IG, Sanderson CJ, Garson OM, Lopez AF, Vadas MA. Interleukin-5 is at 5q31 and is deleted in the 5q- syndrome. *Blood* 1988;**71**:1150.

14 Young Y–C, Kovacic S, Kriz R, Wolf S, Clark SC, Wellems TE, Nienhuis A, Epstein N. The human genes for GM-CSF and IL3 are closely linked in tandem on chromosome 5. *Blood* 1988;**71**:958.

15 D'Eustachio P, Brown M, Watson C, Paul WE The. IL4 gene maps to chromosome 11, near the gene encoding I13 *J. Immunol.* 1988;**141**:3067.

16 Bond MW, Shrader B, Mosmann TR, Coffmann RL. A mouse T cell product that preferentially enhances IgA production. II. Physicochemical characterization. *J. Immunol.* 1987;**139**:3691.

17 McKenzie DT, Filutowicz HI, Swain SI, Dutton RW. Purification and partial sequence analysis of murine B cell growth factor II (interleukin 5). *J. Immunol.* 1987;**139**:2661.

18 Lopez AF, Begley CG, Williamson DJ, Warren DJ, Vadas MA, Sanderson CJ. Murine eosinophil differentiation factor: An eosinophil-specific colony-stimulating factor with activity for human cells. *J. Exp. Med.* 1986;**163**:1085.

19 Strath M, Sanderson CJ. Detection of eosinophil differentiation factor and its relationship to eosinophilia in *Mesocestoides corti*-infected mice. *Exp. Hematol.* 1986;**14**:16.

20 Clutterbuck EJ, Sanderson CJ. Human eosinophil production *in vitro* studied by means of murine eosinophil differentiation factor (IL5). *Blood* 1988;**71**:646.

21 Clutterbuck EJ, Hirst EMA, Sanderson CJ. Human Interleukin 5 (IL5) regulates the production of eosinophils in human bone marrow cultures: comparison and interaction with IL1, IL3, IL6 and granulocyte-macrophage colony-stimulating factor. *Blood* 1989;**73**:1504.

22 Wintrobe HM. Variations of leukocytes in disease. In *Clinical Haematology* (Ed. Wintrobe HM), Lea & Febiger, Philadelphia, 1975, p. 128.

23 Herion JC, Glasser RM, Walker RJ, Palmer JG. Eosinophil kinetics in two patients with eosinophilia. *Blood* 1970;**36**:361.

24 Wetzel BK, Horn RG, Spicer S. Fine structural studies on the development of heterophil, eosinophil, and basophil granulocytes in rabbits. *Lab. Invest.* 1967;**16**:349.

25 Scott RE, Horn RG. Fine structural features of eosinophile granulocyte development in human bone marrow. Evidence for granule secretion. *J. Ultrastruct. Res.* 1970;**33**:16.

26 Henderson WR, Chi EY. Ultrastructural characterisation and morphometric analysis of human eosinophil degranulation. *J. Cell. Sci.* 1985;**73**:33.

27 Bainton DF, Farquhar MG. Segregation and packaging of granule enzymes in eosinophilic leukocytes. *J. Cell. Biol.* 1970;**45**:54.

28 Peters M, Rodriguez M, Gleich G. Localisation of human eosinophil granule major basic protein, eosinophil cationic protein, and eosinophil-derived neurotoxin by immunoelectron microscopy. *Lab. Invest.* 1986;**54**:656.

29 Saito H, Hatake K, Dvorak AM, Leiferman KM, Donnenberg AD, Arai N, Ishizaka K, Ishizaka T. Selective differentiation and proliferation of hematopoietic cells induced by recombinant human interleukins. *Proc. Natl. Acad. Sci. USA* 1988;**85**:2288.

30 Lopez AF, Sanderson CJ, Gamble JR, Campbell HD, Young IG, Vadas, MA. Recombinant human interleukin-5 (IL-5) is a selective activator of human eosinophil function. *J. Exp. Med.* 1987;**167**:219.

31 Begley CG, Lopez AF, Nicola NA, Warren DJ, Sanderson CJ. Purified colony stimulating factors enhance the survival of human neutrophils and eosinophils *in vitro*: a rapid and sensitive microassay for colony stimulating factors. *Blood* 1986;**68**:162.

32 Yamaguchi Y, Suda T, Suda J, Eguchi M, Miura Y, Harada N, Tominaga A, Takatsu K. Purified interleukin 5 (IL-5) supports the terminal differentiation and proliferation of murine eosinophilic precursors. *J. Exp. Med.* 1988;**167**:43.

33 Yamaguchi Y, Hayashi Y, Sugama Y, Miura Y, Kasahara T, Kitamura S, Torisu M, Mita S, Tominaga A, Takatsu T, Suda T. Highly purified murine Interleukin 5 (IL-5) stimulates eosinophil function and prolongs in vitro survival. IL-5 as an eosinophil chemotactic factor. *J. Exp. Med.* 1988;**167**:1737.

34 Strath M, Sanderson, CJ. The production and functional properties of eosinophils from bone marrow cultures. *J. Cell Sci.* 1985;**74**:207.

35 Swain S, Dutton RW. Production of a B cell growth promoting activity, (DL)BCGF, from a cloned T cell line and its assay on the BCL_1 B cell tumor. *J. Exp. Med.* 1982;**156**:1821.

36 O'Garra A, Warren DJ, Holman M, Popham AM, Sanderson CJ, Klaus GGB. Interleukin 4 (B cell growth factor II/ eosinophil differentiation factor) is a mitogen and differentiation factor for preactivated murine B lymphocytes. *Proc. Natl. Acad. Sci. USA* 1986;**83**:5228.

37 Coffmann RL, Shrader B, Carty J, Mosmann TR, Bond MA. A mouse T cell product that preferentially enhances IgA production. I. Biologic characterization. *J. Immunol.* 1987;**139**:3685.

38 Murray PD, McKenzie DT, Swain SL, Kagnoff MF. Interleukin 5 and interleukin 4 produced by Peyers Patch T cells selectively enhance immunoglobulin A expression. *J. Immunol.* 1987;**139**:2669.

39 Harriman GR, Kunimoto DY, Elliott JF, Paetkau V, Strober W. The role of IL-5 in IgA B cell differentiation. *J. Immunol.* 1988;**140**:3033.

40 Yokota T, Coffman RL, Hagiwara H, Rennick DM. Takebe Y, Yokota K, Gemmell L, Shrader B, Yang G, Meyerson P, Luh J, Hoy P, Pene J, Briere F, Spits H, Banchereau J, de Vries J, Lee FD, Arai N, Arai K. Isolation and characterisation of lymphokine cDNA clones encoding mouse and human IgA enhanc-

ing factor and eosinophil colony stimulating factor activities: Relationship to interleukin 5. *Proc. Natl. Acad. Sci. USA* 1987;**84**:7388.

41 Beagley KW, Eldridge JH, Kiyono H, Everson MP, Koopman WJ, Honjo T, McGhee JE. Recombinant murine IL-5 induces high rate synthesis in cycling IgA-positive Peyer's patch B cells. *J. Immunol.* 1988;**141**:2035.

42 Matsumoto R, Matsumoto M, Mita S, Hitoshi Y, Ando M, Araki S, Yamaguchi N, Tominaga A, Takatsu K. Interleukin-5 induces maturation but not class switching of surface IgA-positive B cells into IgA-secreting cells. *Immunol.* 1989;**66**:32.

43 Maizel AL, Sahasrabuddhe S, Mehta SR, Morgan L, Lachman L, Ford R. Biochemical separation of human B cell mitogenic factor. *Proc. Natl. Acad. Sci. USA 1982*;**79**:5998.

44 Clutterbuck EJ, Sheilds J, Gordon J, Smith SH, Boyd A, Callard RE, Campbell HD, Young IG, Sanderson CJ. Recombinant human interleukin-5 (IL5) is an eosinophil differentiation factor but has no activity in standard human B cell growth factor assays. *Eur. J. Immunol.* 1987;**17**:1743.

45 Azuma C, Tanabe T, Konishi M, Noma T, Matsuda F, Yaoita Y, Takatsu K, Hammerstrom L, Smith CIE, Severinson E, Honjo T. Cloning of cDNA for human T cell replacing factor (interleukin-5) and comparison with the murine homologue. *Nucleic Acids Res.* 1986;**14**:9149.

46 Dexter TM, Allen TD, Lajtha LG. Conditions controlling the proliferation of haemopoietic stem cells *in vitro J. Cell. Physiol.* 1977; **91**:335.

47 Warren DJ, Moore MAS. Synergism among interleukin 1, interleukin 3 and interleukin 5 in the production of eosinophils from primitive hemopoietic stem cells. *J. Immunol.* 1988;**140**:94.

48 Clutterbuck EJ, Sanderson CJ. The regulation of human eosinophil precursor production by cytokines: a comparison of rhIL1, rhIL3, rhIL5, rhIL6 and rhGMCSF. *Blood.* 1990 (in press).

49 Pene J, Rousset F, Briere F, Chretien I, Wildmann J, Bonnefoy JY, De Vries JE. Interleukin 5 enhances interleukin 4-induced IgE production by normal human B cells. The role of soluble CD23 antigen. *Eur. J. Immunol.* 1988;**18**:929.

4 · Eosinophil chemotactic factors in asthma and allergy

A.B. Kay

Introduction

Eosinophils are a hallmark of IgE-mediated allergic diseases. They infiltrate the tissue in large numbers in the skin, nose and bronchi after allergen challenge in sensitized atopic subjects. Many appear to be degranulated and it is believed that eosinophil products, particularly granule-associated basic proteins and membrane-derived lipids may be directly responsible for tissue damage (especially epithelial shedding and mucus hypersecretion, which is characteristic of allergic inflammation at mucosal surfaces). Over the past few years several groups have studied the phenomenon of eosinophil activation, both *in vitro* and *in vivo*. The *in vitro* experiments have attempted to increase our knowledge of the eosinophil's repertoire in terms of its responsiveness to pharmacological mediators, particularly those acting through receptors for IgE (FcεRII), IgG (Fc) and complement. The *in vivo* clinical studies were undertaken to provide evidence that eosinophil activation (as shown by the presence of secreted granule products) were related to clinical manifestations and that this in turn might offer further insight into pathogenetic mechanisms, particularly in allergy and asthma.

Over the past decade or so several groups have studied the heterogeneity of human peripheral blood eosinophils. In particular it is now appreciated that cells obtained from patients with hypereosinophilia are metabolically more active than normal eosinophils [1] and separate into low, as well as normal, density cells after centrifugation on Percoll or Metrizamide gradients [2–4]. It is now clear that at least a proportion of these low density cells represent a subpopulation of activated cells. For instance, in the same individual low density cells have increased expression of Fcγ [3] and Fcε receptors [5], are more cytotoxic for opsonized helminthic *in vitro* [6], produce more leukotriene (LT)C_4 than normodense cells after incubation with IgG-coated beads [7] and, in general, respond more vigorously in chemotaxis [8]. Low density cells also showed complete or partial loss of the crystalline granule core and in this sense probably correspond to the vacuolated cells previously observed in peripheral blood from patients with the hypereosinophilic syndrome [9]. In the tissues activated cells can be recognized by a monoclonal antibody (EG2) which distinguishes between the storage and secreted forms of the eosinophil cationic protein (ECP) [10].

The T-cell dependence of control of eosinophilia in rodents has been recognized since the early 1970s and there is now a sizeable literature on eosinophil maturation and activation by various cytokines [reviewed in 11]. It has been shown that tumour necrosis factor (TNF), granulocyte/macrophage-colony stimulating factor (GM-CSF), interleukin-3 (IL-3) and interleukin-5 (IL-5) can augment eosinophil function in a number of ways including enhanced cytotoxic capacity, upregulation of membrane markers and increased metabolic activity [12,13]. In our experience resting human eosinophils, unlike neutrophils, respond weakly in directional locomotion (chemotaxis) to a wide range of cytokines including IL-5, even when tested over a wide concentration range [14]. In contrast, platelet-activating factor (PAF) is a potent eosinophil chemoattractant and, as described below, activates eosinophils to a comparable degree to LTB_4. Furthermore, a variety of physiological stimuli lead to relatively large amounts of both PAF and LTC_4 generation by eosinophils.

PAF and eosinophil chemotaxis

Platelet-activating factor (1-O-alkyl-2-acetyl-*sn*-glycero-3-phosphocholine) is a potent inflammatory mediator with a wide range of biological activities [reviewed in 15]. In human tissues these activities include platelet aggregation and secretion, bronchoconstriction and induction of non-specific bronchial hyperreactivity, leucocyte chemotaxis, modulation of cellular immune functions and inflammatory changes in the skin.

There is comparatively little information on eosinophil activation by PAF. In a previous study we showed that PAF induced directional locomotion of eosinophils, in a time- and dose-dependent fashion, at concentrations from 10^{-5} to 10^{-8} M; lyso-PAF had minimal activity over the same dose range [8]. When PAF was compared with several other documented chemoattractants for eosinophil chemotaxis the rank order of potency (using optimal eosinophilotactic concentrations) was PAF $\geqslant$ C5a $>$ $C5a_{Des\ arg}$ = LTB_4 $>$ FMLP (14). In fact, compared with PAF the eosinophil locomotory responses to LTB_4, histamine and the valyl and alanyl eosinophil tetrapeptides were negligible [8].

We recently established that PAF-induced eosinophil locomotion can be inhibited by a specific PAF antagonist derived from *Ginkgo biloba* (BN 52021) [16]. In response to an optimal concentration of PAF (10^{-6} M) the drug was significantly more potent ($p < 0.001$) in inhibiting eosinophil as compared with neutrophil locomotion (Fig. 4.1). These inhibitory effects were observed in a dose-dependent manner with an IC_{50} of 7.0 ($\pm$2.2)$\times 10^{-6}$ M and 2.3 ($\pm$0.2)$\times 10^{-5}$ M, for eosinophils and neutrophils, respectively. Sodium cromoglycate, nedocromil sodium, salbutamol and dexamethasone (preincubated with cells for up to 6 h) had no effect. Inhibition by BN 52021 was specific for PAF, in that it had no effect on chemotaxis induced by either LTB_4, *N*-formyl-methionyl-leucyl-phenylalanine (FMLP) or a purified human mononuclear cell-derived neutrophil chemotactic factor. BN 52021 also inhibited the specific binding of [^{3}H]-PAF (10^{-8} M) to eosinophils and neutrophils, in a concentration-dependent

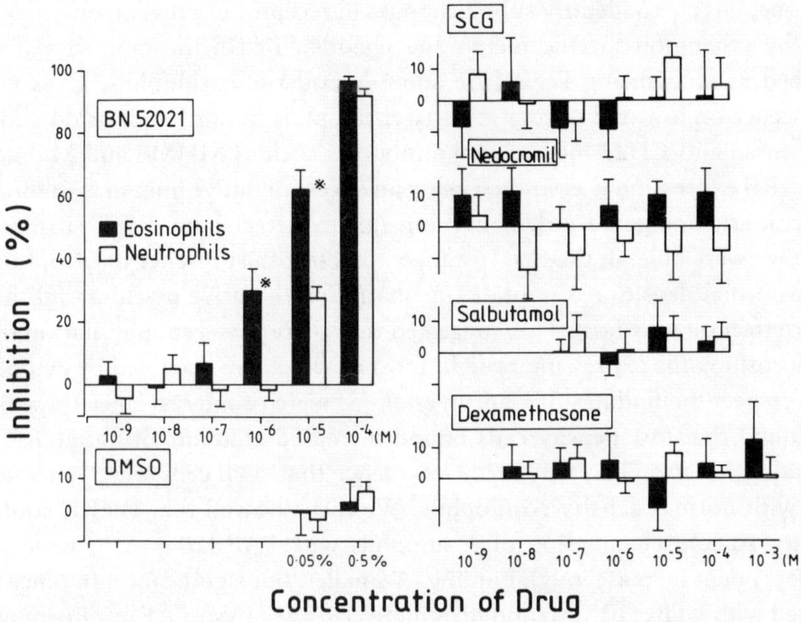

Fig. 4.1. Effects of BN 52021, sodium cromoglycate, nedocromil sodium, salbutamol and dexamethasone on PAF-induced (10^{-6}M) eosinophil (closed bar) and neutrophil (open bar) chemotaxis. Drugs were added to both upper and lower chemotaxis chambers at the beginning of the chemotaxis assay. Diluent of BN 52021, HBSS or RPMI containing equivalent concentrations of DMSO, did not influence the chemotaxis significantly. Each point represents the mean ±SEM of 3–10 experiments. *Significant ($p < 0.001$) differences between the inhibition of eosinophil and neutrophil chemotaxis. (Reproduced from Kurihara *et al. J. Allergy Clin. Immunol.* [16].)

fashion. These results suggest that BN 52021 has potential as an anti-inflammatory agent in conditions associated with PAF-induced accumulation of neutrophils and eosinophils.

PAF and eosinophil membrane receptors

Activation of eosinophils by PAF has been studied in a variety of systems. For instance, PAF (at an optimal concentration of 10^{-7} M) gave dose- and time-dependent increases in the expression of membrane receptors as measured by IgE, IgG and complement rosettes on normal density eosinophils [17]. At 10^{-5} M histamine also produced a small, but significant, percentage enhancement of eosinophil IgE- and IgG-rosettes. In contrast, FMLP (10^{-8} M) enhanced IgG-, but not IgE-dependent, rosettes. In all instances, rosette enhancement was maximal at 30 min after incubation with the activating agent, although still significantly above baseline at 60 min. These findings were extended using flow cytometry (since rosetting is essentially a semi-quantitative technique, unable to identify subtle changes in receptor expression and may be influenced by other non-specific membrane ligands). BB10, the monoclonal antibody described as recognizing FcεRII on some hypodense eosinophils, gives very weak fluorescence on low and normal density eosinophils in our hands as do a number of documented anti-CD23 monoclonal antibodies such as MHM6 and Mab25. Therefore FcεRII expression was studied using an excess of native human myeloma IgE and a fluorescein-conjugated polyclonal anti-IgE to detect bound IgE [18]. Using this system we were able, in the first instance, to detect the presence of cytophilic IgE on resting normal density eosinophils (incubation with native myeloma IgE having no further effect on anti-IgE). This suggested that there was a subpopulation of normal density eosinophils expressing FcεRII, most of which are occupied by cytophilic IgE. In this respect the findings of Capron *et al.* [5] were of interest since these investigations found that low density cells bound increased amounts of native IgE without stimulation *in vitro*. This was further evidence that such cells were 'activated' compared with normal density eosinophils. We then showed that FcεRII could be upregulated since preincubation of eosinophils with PAF (10^{-7} M) gave a time- and dose-dependent increase in IgE binding. A smaller, but significant difference was also observed with LTB_4 (10^{-7} M) and histamine (10^{-5} M). Lyso-PAF or diluent alone had no effect at any of the concentrations used. In time-course studies PAF and LTB_4 gave significant increases in IgE binding after 5 min preincubation, with optimal effect at 30 min.

The complement receptors CR1 and CR3 were also studied on normal density eosinophils using monoclonal antibodies; CR1 is expressed in low numbers but CR3 is expressed in greater density and gives very bright fluorescence. When stimulated, normal density eosinophils showed enhanced expression of CR1 and CR3 in response to PAF but not lyso-PAF in a time- and concentration-dependent fashion similar to that of FcεRII. In Fig. 4.2 upregulation of CR3 on eosinophils and neutrophils by PAF is shown using two-colour flow cytometry. Both cells express similar amounts of CR3 but cytofluorimetry allows eosinophils to be distinguished from neutrophils by their differential expression of Fcγ receptors. Neutrophils express FcγRII (CD32) and FcγRIII (CD16) while eosinophils only express FcγRII [A. Hartnell, unpublished observations].

The effector function of eosinophils, as measured by their ability to adhere to and kill appropriately-opsonized helminthic targets, *in vitro*, was also enhanced by prior stimulation of cells with PAF [17]. Using preparations of IgG- and IgE-rich fractions of immune serum PAF (at an optimal dose of 10^{-8} M) but not lyso-PAF, produced 185, 106 and 100% enhancement of eosinophil cytotoxicity against schistosomula of *Schistosoma mansoni* coated with IgE, IgG and complement, respectively. Leukotriene B_4 also enhanced killing by eosinophils of larvae coated with IgE (95%) and IgG (70%). In contrast, FMLP (optimal dose of 10^{-7} M), enhanced the IgG-(56%) but not IgE-dependent cytotoxicity. This was in contrast to histamine which enhanced the

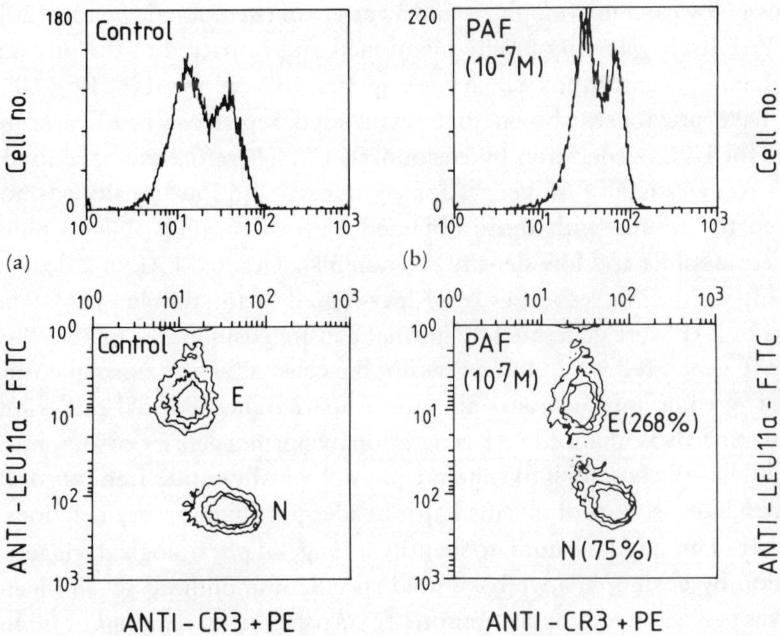

Fig. 4.2. Histograms of relative CR3 fluorescence (horizontal axis) against cell number (vertical axis) of a mixture of eosinophils and neutrophils incubated in either the absence (a), or presence of PAF (10^{-7} M) (b). The accompanying contour plots show the patterns of dual staining of the cell mixture (green fluorescence: vertical axis; red fluorescence: horizontal axis). Neutrophils stained with both monoclonal antibodies (anti-CR3 and anti-Leu 11b) whereas eosinophils staining only with anti-CR3. The enhancement of CR3 expression by PAF was 268% for eosinophils and 75% for neutrophils.

IgE- (77%) but not IgG-dependent *in vitro* killing, albeit at a higher concentration of 10^{-5} M [19]. These studies, which have used a combination of quantitative (i.e. flow cytometry) and functional assays, indicate that various mediators of hypersensitivity can activate human eosinophils *in vitro*, via CR3 and FcεRII. Platelet-activating factor appears to be particularly effective in this respect and since this agent has such a wide range of properties relevant to allergic inflammation it may play a key role in IgE-related inflammatory responses both in allergy and acute immune reactions against helminthic parasites.

PAF and LTC_4 generation by human eosinophils

PAF has been shown to be generated by several human cell types including macrophages, neutrophils, mast cells, and endothelial cells after a variety of physiologic and non-physiologic stimuli. Platelet-activating factor production by eosinophils, however, has been less well documented. One report describes activation of acetyl transferase and acetyl hydrolase (enzymes involved in PAF generation and breakdown respectively) by calcium ionophore and a variety of chemotactic factors [20]. Generation of PAF itself was only briefly mentioned and restricted to the measurement of extracellular concentrations which were apparently very small (< 1 pg/10^6 cells).

We have previously shown that IgG-coated Sepharose beads are an effective stimulus for LTC_4 generation by eosinophils [7]. Therefore we have used the same stimulus to investigate PAF generation by normal and low density eosinophils and compared the results with those obtained with neutrophils. Neutrophils, normal density eosinophils and low density eosinophils generated PAF in a dose- and time-dependent manner in response to an IgG-coated bead stimulus [21]. The greatest amounts of PAF were generated by normal density eosinophils. In all cell types most of the PAF generated was retained within the cells, although normal eosinophils released a greater proportion into the supernatant. Formyl-methyionyl-leucyl-phenylalanine also enhanced PAF generation by normal density eosinophils. Thus the eosinophil has the potential to generate physiologically active amounts of PAF and is therefore a likely source of this mediator in allergic inflammatory reactions.

As part of an ongoing study to identify a range of physiological triggers for LTC_4 production by eosinophils we have used specific immobilized IgG/antigen immune complexes to elicit mediator generation [22]. An extract of *Aspergillus fumigatus* was covalently coupled to Sepharose beads and incubated with the IgG fraction of immune serum from patients with allergic bronchopulmonary aspergillosis (ABPA). These beads elicited generation of 7.72 ± 1.7 pmol LTC_4/10^6 eosinophils as compared with 0.73 ± 0.19 pmol/10^6 cells after eosinophils were incubated with beads treated with IgG from normal non-immune serum. The maximum antibody-dependent release achieved represented approximately 20% of that induced by the calcium ionophore (A23187). Grass pollen–specific IgG antibody/antigen complexes, in combination with Sepharose beads, also triggered generation of LTC_4 immunoreactive material. An IgE myeloma protein, coupled to Sepharose beads, was a weak stimulus of LTC_4 generation by low density cells. However, clearer evidence of IgE-dependent generation of LTC_4 from eosinophils was obtained using opsonized, formalin-fixed shistosomula (Sch) of *S. mansoni* (Table 4.1) [23]. Schistosomula were coated with either IgE or IgG fractions from immune serum separated by FPLC (Polyanion SI-17 column). IgE-rich fractions were identified by parasite-specific RAST and contaminating IgG removed by protein A adsorption. IgG-rich fractions were tested by specific ELISA and confirmed by adsorption on a *Staphylococcus aureus* protein A affinity column. Low density eosinophils, incubated with live or fixed Sch coated with unfractionated immune serum released 16.5 ± 3.5 and 11.7 ± 2.7 pmol of LTC_4/10^6 cells respectively. This is compared with 80 ± 24 and 9.9 ± 1 pmol in the presence of A23187 and IgG-coated beads, respectively. Fixed Sch coated with purified IgE and IgG fractions evoked the release of 7.6 ± 0.4 and 6.0 ± 0.1 pmol of LTC_4 respectively per 10^6 low density eosinophils. Adsorption of IgE on an anti-IgE column abolished the IgE-dependent release of LTC_4 while IgG-dependent generation was removed by protein

Table 4.1. IgE- and IgG-mediated LTC_4 release from, and cytotoxicity of, low density human eosinophils. Eosinophils were incubated with opsonized schistosomula of *S. mansoni* (formalin-fixed for LTC_4 release and live for killing assay). Larvae were coated with untreated immune (anti-*Schistosoma*) serum or FPLC-fractionated IgG- and IgE-rich pools. Parasite-specific IgG and IgE were measured by ELISA and RAST, respectively. IgG-depletion was achieved by adsorption on a protein A column; IgE was removed by an anti-IgE affinity columns

	Specific anti-*Schistosoma*		Hypodense eosinophils	
Opsonin	IgG-ELISA (OD units)	IgE-RAST (% binding)	LTC_4 release (pmol/10^6 cells)	Cytotoxicity (% kill)
Unfractionated immune serum	8.4	36	15±4	82±5
IgG-rich fractions, untreated	6.8	0	6.0±0.1	40±2
IgG-rich fractions+protein A	0.1	0	0.1±0.1	9.4±4
IgG-rich fractions+anti-IgE	6.0	0	5.6±0.3	35±3
IgE-rich fractions, untreated	7.0	35	7.8±0.4	31±1
IgE-rich fractions+protein A	0.18	32	5.5±0.4	30±1.5
IgE-rich fractions+anti-IgE	6.4	0	0.25±0.1	11±2

A, but not anti-IgE adsorption. Thus the release of LTC_4 from eosinophils via IgE-dependent mechanisms following adherence to a helminth may aid in understanding the functional role of the FcεRII in allergy and immunity to helminths.

Clinical studies on eosinophils, allergic inflammation and the late-phase reaction

Our group has also been concerned with attempts to provide direct evidence that eosinophils and their products play a role in tissue damage associated with allergic inflammation. One approach is to identify eosinophil granule products (as an index of activation) in tissues and body fluids and to relate such findings to clinical symptoms. An excellent model of allergen-induced inflammation is the late-phase reaction (LPR).

There have been a number of hypotheses that have sought to relate inflammatory cell infiltrates in LPRs to the subsequent clinical response. Early work suggested that immune complex deposition was important [24], but these claims have not been substantiated and, furthermore, the development or non-appearance of LPRs cannot be predicted from plasma levels of allergen-specific IgG, IgA and IgM. Indeed, allergen-specific IgG appears to attenuate the size of the cutaneous LPR rather than augment it [25]. The ability of $F(ab')_2$ fractions of anti-IgE to elicit LPRs in normal human skin [26] suggested that the LPR was entirely mast-cell-dependent, with cellular infiltration being secondary to the release of mast-cell-derived chemotactic factors. However, the recognition that receptors for IgE (FcεRII) exist on macrophages [27], eosinophils [28], platelets [29] and T-lymphocytes [30] suggests that other cell types may be involved in IgE-mediated reactions. Moreover, drugs such as salbutamol, which are effective mast-cell stabilizers, do not prevent the development of the LPR [31]. On the other hand, corticosteroids, which are extremely effective anti-inflammatory agents, do not influence the immediate allergic response (when given immediately prior to allergen challenge), but are very effective at blocking LPRs in the skin, nose and lung (32).

Eosinophils and cutaneous late-phase reactions. Late-phase allergic reactions provoked either by specific allergen or by anti-IgE are associated with an intense inflammatory cell infiltrate consisting of eosinophils, neutrophils and mononuclear cells [26,33,34]. In man, late-phase reactions (i.e. the delayed in time response observed 3–9 h after allergen administration) are seen in the lungs, nose, skin and conjunctiva. Although there has been a longstanding debate regarding the frequency of occurrence of the late-phase reaction, it now seems likely that LPRs can be elicited in all sensitized individuals and animals, provided enough allergen is administered. This view is based firstly on studies using intradermal injection of anti-IgE in non-atopic volunteers [26] and secondly on recent work in which we have shown that cutaneous LPRs could be elicited in all atopic subjects, provided sufficient allergen was injected [35]. However the magnitude of the late-phase skin reaction clearly varies considerably between individuals following weal and flare responses of similar size [26,33,35].

It has been appreciated for some time that in the late-phase skin reaction, in addition to eosinophils and neutrophils, there is a rich infiltration of mononuclear cells [33,34]. Since it is now clear that T-cell products regulate the production and activation of eosinophils, it seemed reasonable to hypothesize that there may be an appreciable T-cell component of the LPR, at least in the skin, and that this in turn might be related to the intense eosinophilia.

Late-phase skin reactions were induced in subjects with atopic rhinitis by intradermal injection of allergen extracts. Three groups of subjects were used, in whom biopsies were taken after 6, 24 and 48 h respectively. The groups were well matched for age and sex and the size of the weal and LPRs were comparable in all three groups. Six-micrometre thick cryostat sections were cut, fixed in acetone and methanol (50:50) and stained with monoclonal antibodies using the alkaline phosphatase anti-alkaline phosphatase (APAAP) technique. Numerous activated eosinophils were present at the site of allergen challenge as indicated by staining with the monoclonal antibody EG2. These cells and their debris persisted for up to 48 h [36]. T-lymphocytes were also attracted to the cutaneous LPRs: substantial numbers were present by 6 h and T-lymphocytes persisted for up to 48 h. The mean numbers of cells stained with each of the monoclonal antibodies is shown in Table 4.2. The majority of the infiltrating T-lymphocytes CD4+ and the infiltration appeared to be specific in that the CD4+/CD8+ ratio of cells in the skin differed substantially from that measured in the blood. A small number of cells expressed the IL-2 receptor, providing evidence of T-cell activation. Supporting this observation, there was increased expression of HLA-DR by endothelial cells and of CD4 antigen by epidermal Langerhans cells, changes which are thought to be mediated by the T-cell product, interferon-γ [37,38].

Table 4.2. The numbers of infiltrating activated T-lymphocytes and eosinophils in allergen-induced late-phase skin reactions

mAb	Mean cells/field 6 h	24 h	48 h	(Highest control)
CD3	17.42**	13.27*	10.98**	(5.69)
CD4	11.08*	11.45**	6.70*	(4.72)
IL-2R	0.18 NS	0.28*	0.39*	(0.10)
CD8	2.62 NS	2.03 NS	1.52 NS	(1.22)
EG2	14.82****	8.31**	7.90**	(0.64)

Mean number of positively stained cells/field in each group of subjects. Statistical comparisons by Student's *t*-test ($^*p < 0.05$, $^{**}p < 0.01$, $^{****}p < 0.0001$).

Linear regression analysis showed a correlation between the diameter of the LPR (measured at 6 h) and the number of activated eosinophils at 48 h ($r = 0.61$, $p = 0.05$). There was no clear association of LPR size with any of the T-cell subsets but there was a strong association between the number of CD4+ T-cells and the number of activated eosinophils at 24 h ($r = 0.94$, $p < 0.001$) with a similar, but statistically non-significant trend at 48 h ($r = 0.54$). These findings suggest that CD4+ T-lymphocytes and their products, together with eosinophils and their mediators contribute to the pathogenesis of chronic allergic inflammation.

There are several important issues raised by these experiments in terms of the expression of allergic responses. Firstly, there is the question whether activated T-lymphocytes play a role in ongoing chronic allergic diseases (including extrinsic asthma); secondly, the possibility that T-lymphocytes play a part in recruiting granulocytes to sites of allergic inflammation; and finally, the possibility that granulocytes, once recruited, may be activated locally by lymphokines and thereby acquire increased inflammatory potential.

Eosinophils and late-phase asthmatic reactions. In symptomatic allergic asthmatics the numbers of eosinophils in bronchoalveolar lavage (BAL) (in the baseline, 'resting', state) was significantly higher than in asymptomatic asthmatics, hayfever sufferers and normal non-atopic individuals [39]. Similar increases were found in the concentrations of the eosinophil major basic protein (MBP), a major secretory product of activated eosinophils (Fig. 4.3). Furthermore, there were significant correlations between MBP concentrations and (a) the degree of non-specific hyperresponsiveness, (b) the number of shed epithelial cells in BAL, and (c) the BAL eosinophil counts. These findings supported the hypothesis that activated eosinophils release MBP (and presumably other basic proteins from the crystalloid granule), which destroys epithelial cells and in turn accentuates bronchial hyperreactivity.

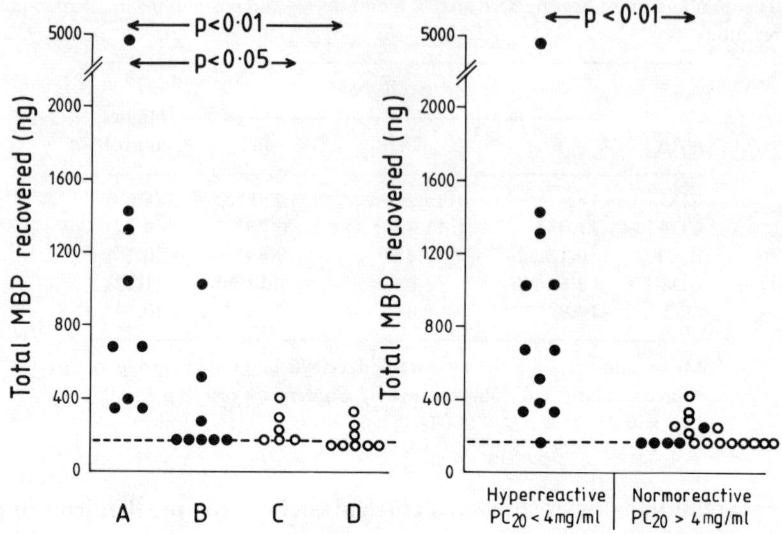

Fig. 4.3. Amount of MBP (ng) recovered from the BAL in four groups of subjects (A, symptomatic asthmatics; B, asymptomatic asthmatics; C, hayfever sufferers; D, non-atopic normal controls) and comparison between hyperreactive and normoreactive subjects. The dotted lines represent amounts below the sensitivity of the assay. (●) Asthmatics, (○) controls. (Reproduced from Wardlaw AJ *et al., Am. Rev. Respir. Dis.* [38].)

Bronchoalveolar lavage studies of the human late asthmatic reaction have also revealed the presence of significantly increased numbers of eosinophils during the late response, whereas relatively modest increases were seen in single early responders [40]. In a recent study we measured the total and differential cell counts, histamine, LTB_4 and LTC_4, immunoglobulins, complement (C), eosinophil-derived basic proteins, and monocyte complement rosettes (MCR) in BAL 6 h after challenge with either antigen (Ag) or diluent (D) control in seven patients with antigen-induced single early reactions (SER), and seven with dual (early- and late-phase) responses. In both groups the total cell counts in BAL were similar, irrespective of whether they were challenged with Ag or D. However, in LPR there were significant increases in lymphocytes, neutrophils and eosinophils, and significant decreases in the percentage of lung mast-cells (Fig. 4.4). MBP and eosinophil-derived neurotoxin (EDN) increased in four out of five subjects with dual responses and most of the patients with SER. Bronchoalveolar lavage histamine concentrations increased in five out of seven patients with dual responses. There were no consistent changes in LTB_4 concentrations in either the LPR or SER groups between D and Ag days; however a small but significant increase in LTC_4 was observed in the LPR group. Concentrations of IgG, IgA, IgM, IgE, C3 and albumin did not differ significantly. The percentage of MCRs also increased significantly ($p < 0.05$) in LPR, but not in SER. These findings support the hypothesis

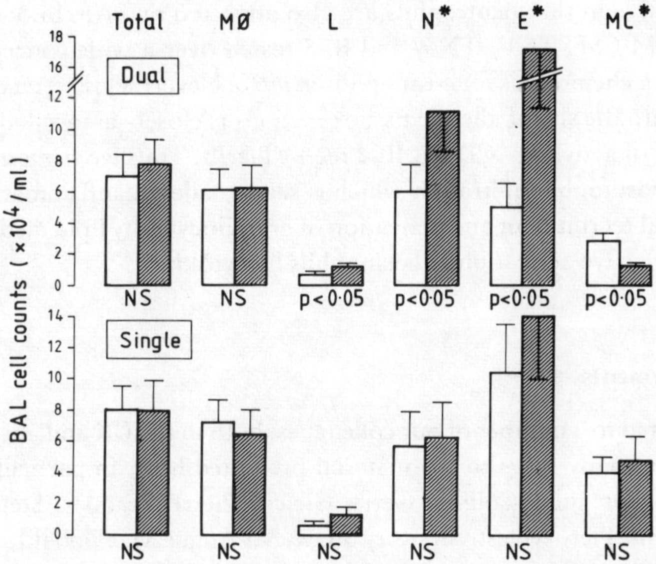

Fig. 4.4. Leucocyte and mast-cell counts in BAL after diluent (□) and antigen (■) challenge in subjects with either dual reactions or single early reactions 6 h following antigen or diluent provocation. The data represent the means and standard errors ($n = 7$). Statistically significant differences 'within groups' (Wilcoxon matched-pair test) are shown. 'Between group' differences (Mann–Whitney *U* test) were not significant (NS). $^{*}\times 10^2$/ml.

that eosinophils and their products play a role in tissue injury in LPR and that eosinophil infiltration may be associated with macrophage activation.

Our recent work also supports the hypothesis that T-cell subsets may be involved in the expression of the late-phase asthmatic reaction in man. Relative increases in CD8+ cells in BAL were seen in single early responders, as compared with late-phase responders [41]. One other study has addressed this area, using segmental bronchial challenge via the fibreoptic bronchoscope in late responders, and demonstrated a selective increase in CD4+ cells in lavage fluid 48 h after challenge [42]. These findings are also consistent with the reported decrease in CD4+ cells in the peripheral blood following allergen inhalation [42] and suggest a selective recruitment and retention of CD4+ T-lymphocytes in the lungs during the late asthmatic reaction.

Summary

Our studies indicate that human eosinophils can be activated in terms of upregulation of surface receptors, increased membrane lipid generation and enhanced cytotoxicity, by a variety of pharmacological mediators through IgE-, IgG- and complement-dependent pathways. Platelet-activating factor is an impressive activator of eosinophil function and is the most potent chemotactic mediator for eosinophils so far described.

It is not selective in that neutrophils are also attracted by PAF. In our experiments, IL-1, IL-2, GM-CSF, TNF, IFN-γ and IL-5 tested over a wide concentration range gave very weak chemotaxis for eosinophils *in vitro*. Nevertheless *in vivo* infiltration of eosinophils into the site of allergic tissue reactions is closely associated with the local accumulation of activated (CD4+, IL-2 rec+) T-cells. Thus we suggest therefore that the selective eosinophil infiltration which is seen in allergic inflammation may result from the initial recruitment and activation of granulocytes by lipid mediators, and the subsequent selective activation of eosinophils by cytokines.

Acknowledgements

We are indebted to a number of our colleagues, both in the UK and abroad, who have contributed in many ways to the material presented here. In particular we wish to acknowledge Drs John Collins, Gerry Gleich, Pierre Braquet, Stephen Durham, Robyn O'Hehir, Piero Maestrelli, Rory Shaw, Mr Angus MacDonald and Miss Dawn Shepherd. This work was supported by the Wellcome Trust (UK), the Medical Research Council (UK), and the Clinical Research Committee of the National Heart and Chest Hospitals, London.

References

1 Bass DA, Grover WH, Lewis J, Szejda P, De Chatelet LR, McCall CE. Comparison of human eosinophils from normals and patients with eosinophilia. *J. Clin. Invest.* 1980;**66**:1558–1564.

2 De Simone D, Donelli G, Mell D, Rosati F, Sorice F. Human eosinophils and parasitic diseases. II. Characterization of two cell fractions isolated at different densities. *Clin. Exp. Immunol.* 1982;**48**:249–255.

3 Winqvist I, Olofsson T, Olsson I, Persson A-M, Hallberg T. Altered density, metabolism and surface receptors of eosinophils in eosinophilia. *Immunology* 1982;**47**:531–539.

4 Prin L, Charon J, Capron M, Gosset P, Taelman H, Tonnel AB, Capron A. Heterogeneity of human eosinophils. II. Variability of respiratory burst activity related to cell density. *Clin. Exp. Immunol.* 1984;**57**:735–742.

5 Capron M, Kusnierz JP, Prin L, Spiegelberg HL, Ovlaque G, Gosset P, Tonnel AB, Capron A. Cytophilic IgE on human blood and tissue eosinophils: detection by flow microfluorometry. *J. Immunol.* 1985;**134**:3013–3018.

6 Capron M, Spiegelberg HL, Prin L, Bennich H, Butterworth AE, Pierce RJ, Aliouaissi M, Capron M. Role of IgE receptors in effector function of human eosinophils. *J. Immunol.* 1984;**132**:462–468.

7 Shaw RJ, Walsh GM, Cromwell O, Moqbel R, Spry CJF, Kay AB. Activated human eosinophils generate SRS-A leukotrienes following physiological (IgG-dependent) stimulation. *Nature* 1985;**316**:150–152.

8 Wardlaw AJ, Moqbel R, Cromwell O, Kay AB. Platelet activating factor. A potent chemotactic and chemokinetic factor for human eosinophils. *J. Clin. Invest.* 1986;**78**:1701–1706.

9 Tai P-C, Spry CJF. Studies on blood eosinophils. I. Patients with a transient eosinophilia. *Clin. Exp. Immunol.* 1976;**24**:415–422.

10 Tai P-C, Spry CJF, Peterson C, Venge P, Olsson I. Monoclonal antibodies distinguish between storage and secreted forms of eosinophil cationic protein. *Nature* 1984;**309**:182–184.

11 Silberstein DS, David JR. The regulation of human eosinophil function by cytokines. *Immunol. Today* 1987;**8**:380–385.

12 Lopez AF, Sanderson CJ, Gamble JR, Campbell HD, Young IG, Vadas MA. Recombinant human interleukin-5 is a selective activator of human eosinophil function. *J. Exp. Med.* 1988;**167**:219–224.

13 Yamaguchi Y, Hayashi Y, Sugama Y, Miura Y, Kasahara T, Kitamura S, Torisu M, Mita S, Tominaga A, Takatsu K, Suda T. Highly purified murine interleukin-5 (IL-5) stimulates eosinophil function and prolongs *in vitro* survival. IL-5 is an eosinophil chemotactic factor. *J. Exp. Med.* 1988;**167**:1737–1742.

14 Kurihara K, Wardlaw AJ, Maestrelli P, Tsai J-J, Kay AB. IL-1, IL-2, TNF, INF-gamma, GM-CSF and PHA-stimulated leukocyte supernatants have negligible eosinophil chemotactic activity compared with platelet activating factor (PAF). *FASEB J.* 1988;**2**:A1449 (abstract 6695).

15 Braquet P, Touqui L, Shen TY, Vargaftig BB. Prospectives in platelet activating factor research. *Pharmacol. Rev.* 1987;**39**:97–145.

16 Kurihara K, Wardlaw AJ, Moqbel R, Kay AB. Inhibition of platelet activating factor (PAF)-induced chemotaxis, and PAF binding to human eosinophils and neutrophils by the specific gingkolide-derived PAF antagonist, BN 52021. *J. Allergy Clin. Immunol.* 1989;**83**:83–90.

17 Moqbel R, Walsh GM, MacDonald AJ, Wardlaw AJ, Kay AB. Activation of human eosinophils by PAF-acether and other inflammatory mediators. *Thorax* 1987;**42**:221 (abstract).

18 Walsh GM, Nagakura T, Moqbel R, Inoue R, Kuriyama T, Kay AB, Iikura Y. Flow cytometric analysis of eosinophil IgE receptor (Fc-epsilon RII); enhancement by platelet activating factor. *Int. Arch. Allergy Appl. Immunol.* 1989;**88**:194–196.

19 Moqbel R, Walsh GM, Nagakura T, MacDonald AJ, Wardlaw AJ, Iikura Y, Kay AB. The effect of platelet activating factor on IgE binding to, and IgE-dependent biological properties of, human eosinophils. *Immunology* (in press).

20 Lee TC, Lenihan DJ, Malone B, Ruddy LL, Wasserman SI. Increased biosynthesis of platelet-activating factor in activated human eosinophils. *J. Biol. Chem.* 1984;**259**:5526–5530.

21 Champion A, Wardlaw AJ, Moqbel R, Cromwell O, Shepherd D, Kay AB. IgG-dependent generation of platelet-activating factor by normal and 'low density' human eosinophils. *J. Allergy Clin. Immunol.* 1988;**81**:207 (abstract 157).

22 Cromwell O, Moqbel R, Fitzharris P, Kurlac L,Harvey C, Walsh GM, Shaw RJ, Kay AB. Leukotriene C_4 generation from human eosinophils stimulated with IgG-*Aspergillus fumigatus* antigen immune complexes. *J. Allergy Clin. Immunol.* 1988;**82**:535–544.

23 Moqbel R, MacDonald AJ, Cromwell O, Kay AB. Release of leukotriene C_4 (LTC_4) from human eosinophils following adherence to IgE- and IgG-coated schistosomula of *Schistosoma mansoni*. *Immunology* 1990;**69**.

24 Pepys J, Turner-Warwick M, Dawson P, Hinson KFW: Arthus (type III) skin test reactions in man. Clinical and immunopathological features. In *Allergology* (Eds Rose B, Richter R, Sehon A, Frankland AW), Excerpta Medica Int Congr Ser Amsterdam; vol. 162, 1968, pp. 221–235.

25 Zetterstrom O. Dual skin test reactions and serum antibodies to subtilisin and *Aspergillus fumigatus* extracts. *Clin. Allergy* 1978;**8**:77–87.

26 Dolovich J, Hargreave FE, Chalmers R, Shier KJ, Gauldie J, Bienenstock J. Late cutaneous allergic responses in isolated IgE-dependent reactions. *J. Allergy Clin. Immunol.* 1973;**52**:38–46.

27 Melewicz FM, Spiegelberg HL. Fc receptors for IgE on a subpopulation of human peripheral blood monocytes. *J. Immunol.* 1980;**125**:1026–1031.

28 Capron M, Capron A, Dessaint J-P, Torpier G, Johansson SGO, Prin L. Fc receptors for IgE on human and rat eosinophils. *J. Immunol.* 1981;**126**:2087–2092.

29 Joseph M, Capron A, Ameisen JC, Capron M, Vorng H, Pancré V, Kusnierz JP, Auriault C. The receptor for IgE on blood platelets. *Eur. J. Immunol.* 1986;**16**:306–312.

30 Prinz JC, Baur X, Ring J, Endres N, Rieker EP. Allergen induced Fc receptors for IgE on human T lymphocytes. *J. Allergy Clin. Immunol.* 1988;**81**:304.

31 Twentyman OP, Holgate ST. Pharmacological modification of the late asthmatic response and effects on circulating inflammatory cells. *J. Allergy Clin. Immunol.* 1987;**79**:150.

32 Booij-Noord H, Orie NG, DeVries K. Immediate and late bronchial obstructive reactions to inhalation of house dust and protective effects of disodium cromoglycate and prednisolone. *J. Allergy Clin. Immunol.* 1971;**48**:344–354.

33 Solley G, Gleich GJ, Jordan R, Schroeter AL. The late phase of the immediate wheal and flare skin reactions: its dependence upon IgE antibodies. *J. Clin. Invest.* 1978;**58**:408–420.

34 Richerson HB, Rajtora D, Penick G, Dick FR, Yoo TJ, Kammermeyer JK, Anuras JS. Cutaneous and nasal allergic responses in ragweed hay fever: lack of clinical and histopathological correlation with late-phase reactions. *J. Allergy Clin. Immunol.* 1979;**64**:67–77.

35 Frew AJ, Kay AB. The pattern of late phase allergic skin reactions in man. *J. Allergy Clin. Immunol.* 1988;**81**:1117–1121.

36 Frew AJ, Kay AB. The relationship between infiltrating CD4+ lymphocytes, activated eosinophils and the magnitude of the allergen-induced late phase cutaneous reaction in man. *J. Immunol.* 1988;**141**:4158–4164.

37 Bevilacqua MP, Pober JS, Majeau GR, Cotran RS, Gimbrone MA Jr. Interleukin 1 induces biosynthesis and cell surface expression of procoagulant activity in human vascular endothelial cells. *J. Exp. Med.* 1984;**160**:618–623.

38 Walsh LJ, Parry A, Scholes A, Seymour GJ. Modulation of CD4 antigen on human gingival Langerhans cells by gamma interferon. *Clin. Exp. Immunol.* 1987;**70**:379–382.

39 Wardlaw AJ, Dunnette S, Gleich GJ, Collins JV, Kay AB. Eosinophils and mast cells in bronchoalveolar lavage in mild asthma: relationship to bronchial hyperreactivity. *Am. Rev. Respir.* 1988;**137**:62–69.

40 De Monchy JGR, Kauffman HF, Venge P, Koeter GH, Jansen HM, Sleuter HJ, DeVries K. Bronchoalveolar eosinophilia during allergen-induced late asthmatic reactions. *Am. Rev. Respir. Dis.* 1985;**131**:373–376.

41 Gonzalez MC, Diaz P, Galleguillos FR, Ancic P, Cromwell O, Kay AB. Allergen-induced recruitment of bronchoalveolar (OKT4) and suppressor (OKT8) cells in asthma. Relative increases in OKT8 cells in single early responders compared with those in late-phase responders. *Am. Rev. Respir. Dis.* 1987;**136**:600–604.

42 Metzger WJ, Zavala D, Richerson HB, Moseley P, Iwamota P, Monick M, Sjoerdsma K, Hunninghake GW. Local allergen challenge and bronchoalveolar lavage of allergic asthmatic lungs. Description of the model and local airway inflammation. *Am. Rev. Respir. Dis.* 1987;**135**:433–440.

43 Gerblich AA, Campbell A, Schuyler M. Changes in T lymphocyte subpopulations after antigenic bronchial provocation in asthmatics. *N. Engl. J. Med.* 1984;**310**:1349–1352.

5 · Interactions between monocytes, macrophages and eosinophils

Caroline J. Howell and T.H. Lee*

Introduction

Arachidonic acid (AA) released from membrane phospholipds after cell activation is metabolized by the cyclooxygenase pathway to prostaglandins and thromboxane and/or by the 5-lipoxygenase pathway to leukotrienes (LT). 5-lipoxygenization of AA that occurs in each type of granulocyte [1–3], results in the generation of LTC_4 and LTB_4. Leukotriene C_4 is the major leukotriene produced by the human eosinophil (EOS), whereas LTB_4 is the major leukotriene produced by the human neutrophil (PMN).

Leukotriene C_4 contracts smooth-muscle and increases vasopermeability [4–6]. It is sequentially converted to the cysteinyl–glycyl and cysteinyl analogues, LTD_4 and LTE_4, which together with LTC_4 constitute the activity termed slow reacting substance of anaphylaxis (SRS–A) [8].

Previous work has demonstrated that human EOS and PMN incubated with supernatants of cultures of lipopolysaccharide (LPS)-stimulated blood mononuclear cells demonstrate enhanced abilities to produce leukotrienes when activated by the calcium ionophore A23187 [8,9]. This enhancement occurred via a permissive effect on phospholipase A_2 activity. The enhancing activity was produced by immunoglobulin-negative, Leu-1 negative, adherent blood mononuclear cells, which were presumed to be monocytes. This activity was shown to be distinct from interleukin-1 (IL-1), interferons (IFN) α and β, granulocyte macrophage-colony stimulating factor (GM-CSF) and tumour necrosis factor (TNF) which also enhance EOS function. The activity may bc similar to that isolated from monocytes of individuals with a moderate eosinophilia [10–12], termed eosinophil activating factor (EAF); EAF is a 40 kD protein of pI 4.4.

Recent results

We have recently extended the studies with monocytes to compare the effects of supernatants derived from alveolar macrophages (AM) isolated from normal and asthmatic subjects to modulate EOS LTC_4 generation. Incubation of EOS with AM supernatants followed by stimulation with A23187 resulted in enhancement of the capacity of EOS

Support: The work was supported in parts by the Wellcome Trust and Asthma Research Council.
*To whom correspondence should be addressed.

to secrete LTC_4. Supernatants derived from AM of asthmatic subjects were more active than those from AM of normal individuals. Enhancement was maximal when EOS were preincubated with a one-sixth dilution of AM supernatants for 5 min at 37°C and were then stimulated with 5 μM A23187 for 15 min. There was an inverse correlation between the percentage enhancement and the A23187-stimulated LTC_4 production in the absence of cytokine ($r = -0.48$, $p < 0.01$). Separation of AM supernatants by size exclusion HPLC using a TSK G 3000 SW column resulted in a peak of enhancing activity which was heat and trypsin sensitive with an estimated molecular size of between 29 000 and 66 000 daltons. Further purification by anion exchange HPLC using a TSK DEAE 5PW column (pH 7.4) resolved the activity into two consistent peaks which eluted at 0.17 and 0.2 M NaCl respectively. Analysis of the fractions from anion exchange for IL-1 and TNF (by bioassay and ELISA respectively), showed that these molecules did not co-elute with the EOS enhancing activity. The major activity which eluted at 0.2 M NaCl following anion exchange was further resolved by reverse-phase HPLC using a C18 Spherisorb ODS column and a slope gradient of 0–100% acetonitrile in 0.1% trifluoroacetic acid as eluting solvent. This demonstrated a single peak of activity which eluted at 41% acetonitrile.

The findings that the activity was an acidic protein of molecular size between 29 000 and 66 000 daltons and which eluted at approximately 40% acetonitrile by RP-HPLC were suggestive of GM-CSF. Specific antibody to GM-CSF completely neutralized the activity whereas anti-G-CSF and pre-immunization serum did not affect the activity. The identity of the activity as GM-CSF was further supported by the finding that preincubation of EOS with recombinant GM-CSF under identical conditions as those already indicated led to an enhancement of LTC_4 generation.

Granulocyte macrophage-colony stimulating factor

This is an acidic glycoprotein of pI 4.5, with a molecular weight of 22 000 daltons, which elutes from size exclusion chromatography columns between 15 000 and 40 000 daltons, depending on the extent of glycosylation. It elutes from DEAE cellulose anion exchange chromatography columns at between 0.1 and 0.2 M NaCl. Granulocyte macrophage-colony stimulating factor is produced from human endothelial cells, fibroblasts and T-cells [13–15]. In addition an eosinophil-stimulating activity that co-purifies with GM-CSF can be isolated from the supernatant of cultured monocytes [16]. Although GM-CSF can be released in the absence of exogenous stimuli, production of this cytokine can be stimulated by IL-1β [15,17], TNF [14,18] and LPS [19,20].

The major biological activity of GM-CSF is to induce the proliferation and differentiation of neutrophilic, eosinophilic and monocytic stem cells [21–24]. Other biological activities of GM-CSF include the prolongation of EOS and PMN [25,26] survival in culture, induction of histamine release from basophils and mast-cells [27,28], enhancement of PGE_2 production from macrophages and the consequent inhibition of IL-2 receptor expression [29], stimulation of the expression of C3bi, Mo1 granulocyte functional antigens 1 and 2 [26] and Leu M5 expression [30]. In addition GM-CSF primes EOS and PMN for enhanced cytotoxic killing [26,31–33], enhanced leukotriene production [33–35] via a permissive effect on arachidonic acid release [35] and enhanced phagocytosis of zymosan [26] and bacteria [36]. The human neutrophil, pretreated with GM-CSF exhibits an increased rate of membrane depolarization [37] and enhanced degranulation and superoxide anion release following stimulation with FMLP C5a des Arg and LTB_4 [26,38,39]. Polymorphonuclear neutrophils have augmented responsiveness towards chemotactic agonists in the presence of GM-CSF [39]. Finally, GM-CSF activates macrophages and neutrophils to produce other cytokines, such as IL-1, TNF, G-CSF and M-CSF [40, reviewed in 41], and activates PBMC to become tumoricidal [42].

Conclusion

We have demonstrated that AM isolated from asthmatic individuals spontaneously produce an activity which enhances the capacity of A23187-activated eosinophils to generate LTC_4. The activity has been identified as GM-CSF. These findings suggest that GM-CSF may play an important role in the amplification of the eosinophilic inflammation which is so characteristic of asthmatic airways.

References

1 Samuelsson B. Leukotrienes; mediators of immediate hypersensitivity reactions and inflammation. *Science* 1983;**220**:568–575.

2 Lewis RA, Austen KF. The biologically active leukotrienes; biosynthesis, metabolism, receptors, functions and pharmacology. *J. Clin. Invest.* 1984;73:889–897.

3 Jorg A, Henderson WR, Murphy RC, Klebanoff SJ. Leukotriene generation by eosinophils. *J. Exp. Med.* 1982;**155**:390–402.

4 Drazen JM, Austen KF, Lewis RA, Clark DA, Goto G, Marfat A, Corey EJ. Comparative airway and vascular activities of leukotrienes C and D *in vivo* and *in vitro*. *Proc. Natl. Acad. Sci. USA* 1980;77:4354–4358.

5 Peck MJ, Piper PJ, Williams TJ. The effects of leukotrienes C_4 and D_4 on the microvascular of guinea-pig skin. *Prostaglandins* 1981;**21**:315–321.

6 Dahlen SE, Bjork J, Hedqvist P, Arfors KE, Hammarstrom S, Lindgren JA, Samuelsson B. Leukotrienes promote plasma leakage and leukocyte adhesion in post capillary venules. *In vivo* effects with relevance to the acute inflammatory response. *Proc. Natl. Acad. Sci. USA* 1981;**78**:3887–3891.

7 Lewis RA, Drazen JM, Austen KF, Clark DA, Corey EJ. Identification of the C(6)-*S*-conjugate of leukotriene A with cysteine as a naturally occurring slow reacting substance of anaphylaxis. (SRS-A). Importance of the 11-*cis*-geometry for biological activity. *Biochem. Biohys. Res. Commun.* 1980;**96**:271–277.

8 Dessein AJ, Lee TH, Elsas P, Ravalese J, Silberstein D, David JR, Austen KF, Lewis RA. Enhancement by monokines of leukotriene generation by human eosinophils and neutrophils stimulated with calcium ionophore A23187. *J. Immunol.* 1986;**136**:3829–3837.

9 Elsas P, Lee TH, Lenzi HL, Dessein AJ. Monocytes activate eosinophils for enhanced helminthotoxicity and increased generation of leukotriene C_4. *Ann. Inst. Pasteur/Immunol.* 1987;**138**:97–116.

10 Thorne KJI, Richardson BA, Veith MC, Tai PC, Spry CJF, Butterworth AE. Partial purification and biological properties of an eosinophil-activating factor. *Eur. J. Immunol.* 1985;**15**:1083–1091.

11 Fitzharris P, Moqbel R, Thorne KJI, Richardson BA, Hartnell A, Cromwell O, Butterworth AE, Kay AB. The effects of eosinophil activating factor on IgG-dependent sulphidopeptide leukotriene generation by human eosinophils. *Clin. Exp. Immunol.* 1986;**66**:673–680.

12 Thorne KJI, Richardson BA, Taverne J, Williamson DJ, Vadas MA, Butterworth AE. A comparison of eosinophil activating factor (EAF) with other monokines and lymphokines. *Eur. J. Immunol.* 1986;**16**:1143–1149.

13 Chan JY, Slamon DJ, Nimer SD, Golde DW, Gasson JC. Regulation of expression of human granulocyte macrophage colony-stimulating factor (GM-CSF) *Proc. Natl. Acad. Sci. USA* 1986;**83**:8669–8673.

14 Munker R, Gasson JC, Ogawa M, Koeffler HP. Recombinant human tumour necrosis factor induces production of granulocyte monocyte colony stimulating factor mRNA and protein from lung fibroblasts and vascular endothelial cells *in vitro*. *Nature* 1986;**323**:79–82.

15 Kaushansky K, Lin N, Adamson JW. Interleukin-1 stimulates fibroblasts to synthesize granulocyte-macrophage and granulocyte colony stimulating factor. Mechanism for the haemopoietic response to inflammation. *J. Clin. Invest.* 1988;**81**:92–97.

16 Vadas M, Nicola N, Lopez AF, Metcalf D, Johnson G, Pereira A. Mononuclear cell-mediated enhancement of granulocyte function in man. *J. Immunol.* 1984;**133**:202–207.

17 Broudy VC, Kanshensky K, Harlan JM, Adamson JW. Interleukin-1 stimulated human endothelial cells to produce granulocyte macrophage-colony stimulating factor and granulocyte-colony stimulating factor. *J. Immunol.* 1987;**139**:464–468.

18 Lu L, Srow EF, Warren DJ, Walker D, Graham CD, Walker EB, Jansen J, Broxmeyer HE. Enhancement of release of granulocyte and granulocyte macrophage-colony stimulating factors from phycohaemagglutinin sorted subsets of human T lymphocytes by recombinant human tumour necrosis factor. Synergism with recombinant human IFN-γ. *J. Immunol.* 1988;**141**:201–207.

19 Metcalf D. *The Hemopoietic Colony Stimulating Factor*. Elsevier Science Publishers, Amsterdam, 1984.

20 Thorens B, Mermod J–J, Vansalli P. Phagocytosis and inflammatory stimuli induce GM-CSF mRNA in macrophages through post-transcriptional regulation. *Cell* 1987;**48**:671–679.

21 Nicola NA, Metcalf D, Johnson GR, Burgess AW. Separation of functionally distinct human granulocyte macrophage-colony stimulating factor. *Blood* 1979;**54**:614–627.

22 Abboud CN, Brennan JK, Barlow GH, Lichtman MA. Hydrophobic adsorption chromatography of colony stimulating activities and erythroid-enhancing activity from the human monocyte-like cell line GCT. *Blood* 1981;**58**:1148–1154.

23 Lee F, Yokota T, Otsuka T, Gemmell L, Larsen N, Luh J, Arai KI, Rennick D. Isolation of cDNA for a human granulocyte macrophage-colony stimulating factor by functional expression in mononuclear cells. *Proc. Natl. Acad. Sci. USA* 1985;**82**:4360–4364.

24 Metcalf D, Begley CG, Johnson GR, Nicola NA, Vadas M, Lopez A, Williamson DJ, Wang EA, Wang CG, Clark SC. Biologic properties *in vitro* of recombinant human granulocyte macrophage-colony stimulating factor. *Blood* 1986;**67**:37–45.

25 Owen WF, Rothenberg ME, Silberstein DR, Gasson JC, Stevens RL, Austen KF, Soberman RJ. Regulation of human eosinophil viability, density and function by granulocyte macrophage-colony stimulating factor in the presence of 3T3 fibroblasts. *J. Exp. Med.* 1987;**166**:129–141.

26 Lopez AF, Williamson DJ, Gamble JR, Begley CG, Harlan JM, Klebanoff SJ, Waltersdorph A, Wong G, Clark SC, Vadas MA. Recombinant human granulocyte macrophage-colony stimulating factor stimulates *in vitro* mature human neutrophil and eosinophil function, surface receptor expression and survival. *J. Clin. Invest.* 1986;**78**:1220–1228.

27 Haak-Frendscho M, Arai N, Arai K–I, Baeza ML, Finn A, Kaplan AP. Human recombinant granulocyte macrophage-colony stimulating factor and interleukin-3 cause basophil histamine release. *J. Clin. Invest.* 1988;**82**:17–20.

28 Dy M, Schneider E, Gastinel L–N, Auffray C, Mermod JJ, Hamburger J. Histamine-producing cell-stimulating activity. A biological activity shared by interleukin-3 and granulocyte macrophage-colony stimulating factor. *Eur. J. Immunol.* 1987;**17**:1234–1248.

29 Hancock WW, Pleau ME, Kobzik L. Recombinant granulocyte macrophage colony-stimulating factor down-regulates expression of IL-2 receptor on human mononuclear phagocytes by induction of prostaglandin. *Eur. J. Immunol.* 1988;**140**:3021–3025.

30 Arnaout MA, Wang EA, Clark SC, Sieff CA. Human recombinant granulocyte macrophage-colony stimulating factor increases cell-to-cell adhesion and surface expression of adhesion-promoting surface glycoproteins on mature granulocytes. *J. Clin. Invest.* 1986;**78**:597–601.

31 Dessein AJ, Vadas MA, Nicola NA, Metcalf D, David JR. Enhancement of human blood eosinophil cytotoxicity by semi-purified eosinophil colony stimulating factor. *J. Exp. Med.* 1982;**156**:90–103.

32 Vadas MA, Nicola NA, Metcalf D. Activation of antibody dependent cell-mediated cytotoxicity of human neutrophils and eosinophils by separate colony stimulating factors. *J. Immunol.* 1983;**130**:795–799.

33 Silberstein DS, Owen WF, Gasson JC, Di Persio JF, Golde DW, Bina JC, Soberman R, Austen KF, David JR. Enhancement of human eosinophil cytotoxicity and leukotriene synthesis by biosynthetic (recombinant) granulocyte macrophage-colony stimulating factor. *J. Immunol.* 1986;**137**:3290–3294.

34 Dahinden CA, Zingg J, Maly FE, de Weck AL. Leukotriene production in human neutrophils primed by recombinant human granulocyte macrophage-colony stimulating factor and stimulated with the complement component C5A and FMLP as second signals. *J. Exp. Med.* 1988;**167**:1281–1295.

35 Di Persio JF, Billing P, Williams R, Glasson JC. Human granulocyte macrophage-colony stimulating factor and other cytokines prime human neutrophils for enhanced arachidonic acid release and leukotriene B_4 synthesis. *J. Immunol.* 1988;**140**:4315–4322.

36 Fleischmann J, Golde DW, Weisbat RH, Gasson JC. Granulocyte macrophage-colony stimulating factor enhances phagocytosis of bacteria by human neutrophils. *Blood* 1986;**68**:708–711.

37 Sullivan R, Griffin JD, Simons ER, Schafer AI, Meshulan T, Fredette JP, Maas AK, Gadenne AS, Leavitt JL, Melnick DA. Effects of recombinant human, granulocyte and macrophage-colony stimulating factors on signal transduction pathways in human granulocytes. *J. Immunol.* 1987;**139**:3422–3430.

38 Kapp A, Zeck-Kapp G, Danner M, Luger TA. Human granulocyte macrophage-colony stimulating factor. An effective direct activator of human polymorphonuclear neutrophilic granulocytes. *J. Invest. Dermatol.* 1988;**91**:49–55.

39 Weisbart RH, Kwan L, Golde DW, Gasson JC. Human GM-CSF primes neutrophils for enhanced oxidative metabolism in response to major physiologic chemoattractants. *Blood* 1987;**69**:18–21.

40 Lindemann A, Riedel D, Oster W, Meuer SC, Blohm D, Mertelsmann RH, Herrman F. Granulocyte macrophage-colony stimulating factor induces interleukin-1 production by human polymorphonuclear neutrophils. *J. Immunol.* 1988;**140**:837–839.

41 Cosman D. Colony-stimulating factors *in vivo* and *in vitro*. *Immunol. Today* 1988;**9**:97–98.

42 Grabstein KH, Urdal DL, Tushinski RJ, Mochizuki DY, Price VL, Cantrell MA, Gillis S, Conlon PJ. Induction of macrophage tumoricidal activity by granulocyte macrophage-colony stimulating factor. *Science* 1986;**232**:506–508.

6 · Interactions between PAF, cytokines, the CD11/18 complex and eosinophil adherence reactions *in vitro*

G.M. Walsh*, Adele Hartnell, R. Moqbel, K. Kurihara and A.B. Kay

Summary

Platelet-activating factor (PAF) and other inflammatory mediators are thought to play an important role in the recruitment and activation of eosinophils to sites of allergic type inflammation. An important *in vivo* event in eosinophil accumulation is their adherence to the endothelial cells lining the blood vessels feeding inflammatory sites. We have investigated some of the mechanisms involved in this process utilizing *in vitro* assays of eosinophil adherence to plasma coated glass (PCG) or human microvascular endothelial cells (HMVEC). Platelet-activating factor, granulocyte/macrophage-colony stimulating factor (GM-CSF) and the recombinant human interleukin-5 (rhIL-5) were investigated for their ability to upregulate eosinophil adhesion to PCG and HMVEC. The role of the CD11/18 family of adhesion molecules in this process was also investigated using a panel of specific monoclonal antibodies.

Introduction

Both helminthic infections and allergic inflammation are associated with a blood and tissue eosinophilia [1]. Following stimulation *in vitro* eosinophils release an array of pre-formed [2] and *de novo* synthesized membrane-derived mediators [3,4]. These products are thought to be important contributory factors in allergic inflammation, e.g. the denudation of the bronchial epithelium in asthma by major basic protein [5]. Furthermore, post-mortem studies have revealed eosinophil accumulation in association with epithelial denudation [6] and a correlation has been demonstrated between the blood eosinophil count and bronchial hyperreactivity [7]. These observations implicate the eosinophil as a primary pro-inflammatory cell.

In vivo leucocyte accumulation is preceded by their adherence to endothelial cells lining the blood vessels, followed by extravasation and migration through tissues to inflammatory sites. A number of *in vitro* studies have demonstrated the involvement of a family of heterodimeric leucocyte cell surface proteins in adhesion reactions with umbilical cord-derived human vascular endothelial cells (HVEC) and a number of synthetic substrates. This leucocyte integrin family consists of three distinct, but

*To whom correspondence should be addressed.

related α sub-units (LFA-1 α, CR3 α and p150,95 α, CD11a, b and c respectively) in a non-covalent association with a common β chain sub-unit (CD18). Their heterodimeric structure and the strong homology at the amino acid level with other cell surface adhesion receptors render these glycoproteins members of the supergene family of integrins [for review see reference 8]. Table 6.1 outlines some of the characteristics and cellular distribution of these receptors. The importance of these receptors is emphasized by the existence of an autosomal recessive heritable disorder designated leucocyte adhesion deficiency (LAD). The leucocytes of these individuals are deficient in expression of the CD11/18 complex, resulting in life-threatening recurrent bacterial infections [for review see reference 9]. A number of distinct adhesion proteins have also been shown to be present on vascular endothelial cells one of which, intercellular adhesion molecule-1 (ICAM-1), is the ligand for LFA-1α [10–12]. It can be assumed that the emigration of eosinophils from blood vessels feeding inflammatory sites must also first require their adhesion to vascular endothelium and that this process is a specific one, reliant upon the presence of eosinophil and endothelial cell adhesion proteins. In a comparative study, we recently investigated phenotypic marker expression by resting human eosinophils, neutrophils and mononuclear cells. CR3 and LFA-1 were found to be present on eosinophils in similar amounts to that of the neutrophil, while p150,95 was only weakly expressed by both cell types [13].

Table 6.1. Characteristics of the CD11/18 family of membrane adhesion proteins

Glycoprotein	Subunits	Function
LFA-1 (CD11a/CD18)	180 kD 95 kD	Leucocyte–endothelial adhesion, T, B and monocyte aggregation, cellular cytotoxicity (NK, K, CTC, ADCC), T-helper responses, blastogenesis
CR3 (CD11b/CD18) (Mac-1)	170 kD 95 kD	iC3b binding, granulocyte phagocytosis, aggregation, chemotaxis and spreading, eosinophil-mediated ADCC
p150,95 (CD11c/CD18)	150 kD 95 kD	iC3b binding, adherence reactions

The membrane-derived phospholipid, PAF has been shown to be the most potent eosinophilotactic agent so far described, although it is not selective for the eosinophil, being an equally potent neutrophil chemoattractant [14]. PAF has been demonstrated to stimulate increased eosinophil adherence to cultured human vascular endothelial cells (HVEC) or plastic plates [15] and to enhance cytotoxicity against opsonized larvae of *Schistosoma mansoni* [16]. In addition, PAF enhanced eosinophil C3b-, IgE- and IgG-dependent rosette formation [17], and has been demonstrated to have effects on cultured human endothelial cells, including shape changes and loss of physical contact [18].

A number of studies have demonstrated that the survival of human peripheral blood eosinophils can be prolonged and their functional properties enhanced; i.e. when co-cultured with human recombinant granulocyte/macrophage-colony stimulating factor (GM-CSF) in the presence of mouse 3T3 fibroblasts [19], or with recombinant human interleukin-3 (rhIL-3) [20]. In addition to their eosinophil differentiating activity on cultured human bone marrow [21], recombinant human rhIL-3 and interleukin-5 (rhIL-5) have also been shown to enhance the effector function of normal density human eosinophils, extend their survival and induce them to become hypodense [20,22,23].

For these reasons we wished to test the effect of the human recombinant cytokines GM-CSF and IL-5 on eosinophil adherence reactions *in vitro* to PCG and human microvascular endothelial cells cultured from human fetal omental fat pad (HMVEC), and to compare their potency with PAF. Furthermore, the role of all the members of the CD11/18 family of adhesion proteins in this process was investigated, using a panel of specific monoclonal antibodies (kindly supplied by Dr T. Springer) in both inhibition assays and flow cytometric analysis.

Eosinophil adherence to PCG and HMVEC

Human eosinophils were purified as previously described [24] and pre-incubated with PAF, lyso-PAF, GM-CSF or rhIL-5 before being allowed to settle onto glass chamber

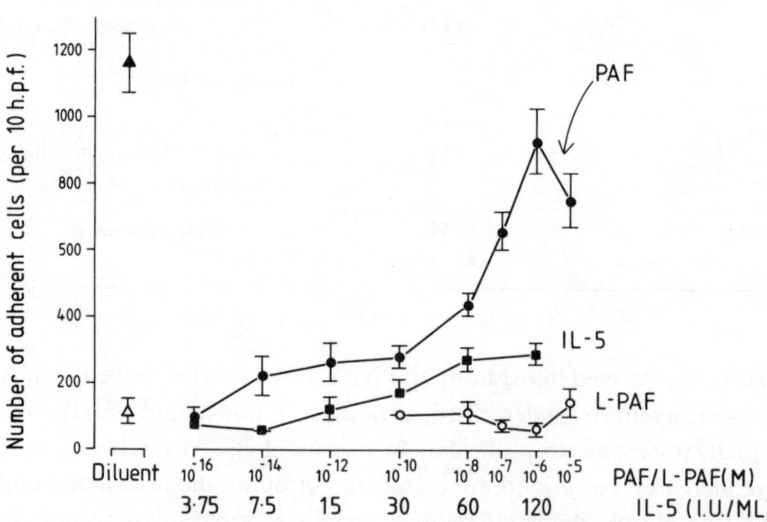

Fig. 6.1. Dose–response of the effect of PAF, L-PAF and IL-5 on eosinophil adherence to plasma coated glass. Each point represents the mean ± SEM of five experiments.

slides pre-coated with 10% pooled human plasma. Following detachment of non-adherent cells by inverting the chambers, the slides were fixed stained and mounted. The numbers of adherent eosinophils in 10 random high power fields (hpf) were counted in a blind fashion.

PAF gave a dose-dependent increase in eosinophil adherence optimal at 10^{-6}M, while IL-5 gave a lower order of enhancement (Fig. 6.1). In addition to the large increase in adherent cell numbers, stimulated eosinophils exhibited striking changes in orientation and polarization, confirming the observations of Lopez *et al.* [22]. Time-course studies revealed that IL-5 had a less rapid effect than PAF (Fig. 6.2), with optimal enhanced adhesion observed at 60 min. Although this time-course is too fast for *de novo* protein synthesis, the recruitment of newly synthesized adhesion receptors to the cell surface as a consequence of RNA translation cannot be excluded. A comparison of the effect of PAF, IL-5 and GM-CSF, on eosinophil and neutrophil adhesion to PCG is shown in Fig. 6.3. IL-2 was also tested and had no effect on either cell type. Generally, baseline and enhanced levels of eosinophil adhesion to PCG were higher than those of the neutrophil; in addition IL-5 had negligible effect on neutrophil hyperadherence. Our observations of the selective effect of IL-5 were extended using cultured HMVEC grown to confluence on glass slides, the adhesion assay was performed as described above. IL-5 gave dose-dependent increases in eosinophil, but not neutrophil adherence to HMVEC (Fig. 6.4). Granulocyte macrophage-colony stimulating factor and PAF, but not lyso-PAF, enhanced both eosinophil and neutrophil adherence to HMVEC.

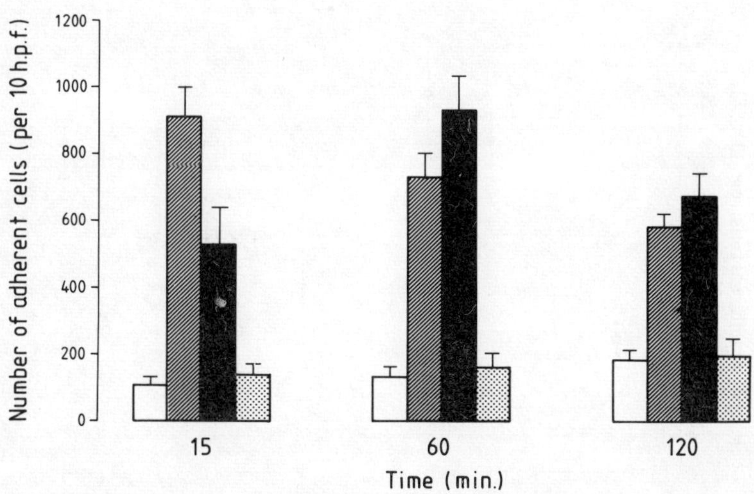

Fig. 6.2. Time-course of the effect of PAF, L-PAF and IL-5 on eosinophil adherence to plasma coated glass. Each point represents the mean ± SEM of four experiments (□) Diluent, (▨) PAF (10^{-6} M), (■) IL-5 (120 IU/ml), (□) L-PAF (10^{-6} M).

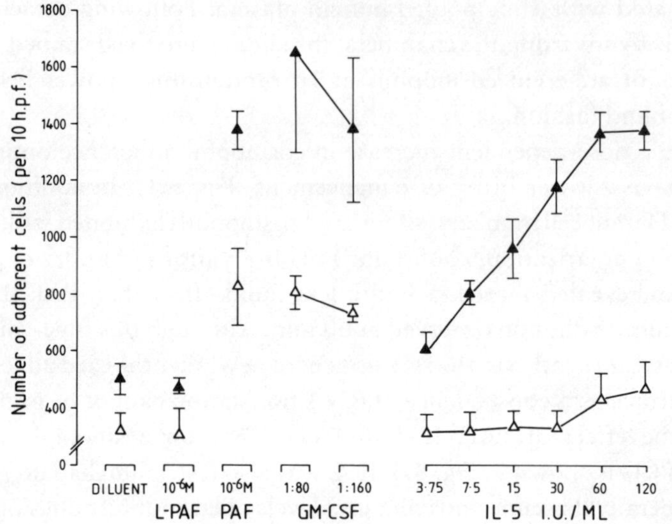

Fig. 6.3. A comparison of eosinophil (▲) and neutrophil (△) adherence with plasma coated glass following stimulation with PAF, L-PAF, GM-CSF and IL-5. Each point represents the mean ± SEM of five experiments.

Human interleukin-5, in addition to stimulating eosinophil proliferation, has been demonstrated to be an activator of human eosinophil, but not neutrophil function [22]. We have observed rhIL-5 to be potent and selective in the enhancement of eosinophil adhesion to PCG and HMVEC. The demonstration of a substance specific

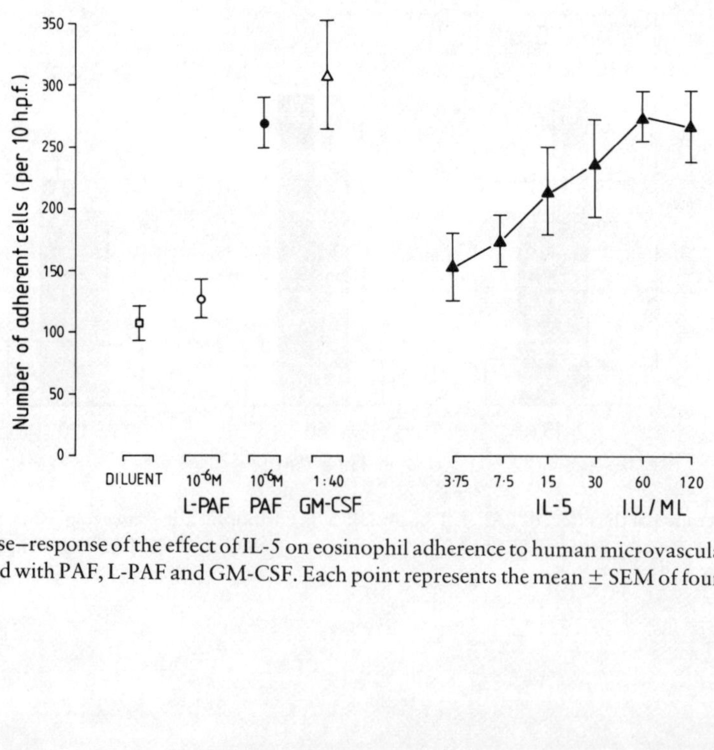

Fig. 6.4. A dose–response of the effect of IL-5 on eosinophil adherence to human microvascular endothelial cells compared with PAF, L-PAF and GM-CSF. Each point represents the mean ± SEM of four experiments.

for eosinophil hyperadherence may have implications for a number of clinical conditions, particularly asthma. Lung biopsies taken from subjects who have died from asthma have revealed the hallmark of this disease, the accumulation of large numbers of eosinophils in and around the airways [25]; however the complex mechanisms responsible for eosinophil accumulation in the asthmatic lung remain to be elucidated. In addition, some cases of lung carcinoma are associated with an eosinophilia [26] and extracted tumour has been demonstrated to produce a substance that preferentially stimulates eosinophil function *in vitro* [27]. Interleukin-5 has, at best, been shown to have very weak eosinophil chemotactic activity [23,28], but may play a role in the selective extravasation of eosinophils into the tissues, where non-specific chemoattractants such as PAF might complete their attraction to inflammatory foci.

CONTRIBUTION OF THE CD11/18 COMPLEX

Neutrophil CR3 expression is known to be upregulated three- to 10-fold following cell stimulation with a number of substances [29,30] as is p150,95 [31]. Additionally, PAF has been shown to enhance neutrophil complement receptor expression [32]. It seems reasonable to assume that upregulation of receptor numbers is responsible for neutrophil hyperadherence, but this does not appear to be the case [33,34]. We observed that as for the neutrophil, eosinophils do not increase LFA-1 or p150,95 expression following PAF-induced stimulation (Fig. 6.4). CR3 showed measurable but insignificant increases in expression after PAF stimulation and with regard to this our data agree with the findings of Kimani *et al.* [15], who utilized an anti-common β-chain mcAb. It seems that eosinophil enhanced adhesion is dependent upon a change in affinity or confirmation, such as 'clustering' in the receptor, the latter appears to be the case for the neutrophil [35] and may be true for the eosinophil. Furthermore, neutrophil CR3 recruited from intracellular pools following cell activation does not appear to be functionally active [36], providing further evidence that hyperadherence by stimulated cells is not dependent upon a simple increase in receptor numbers.

The role of the CD11/18 family of adhesion proteins in the adhesion of eosinophils to PCG and HMVEC was further assessed in inhibition assays using specific mcAbs (Fig. 6.5). Enhanced adhesion PAF (10^{-6}M) for PCG assay or IL-5 (60 IU/ml) for HMVEC assay was significantly inhibited by (ranked in order of potency) anti-CR3, anti-common β-chain and anti-LFA-1. McAbs against p150,95, CD-45, ICAM-1 and the isotype negative control had no measurable inhibitory effect. No significant inhibition by mcAbs of adhesion by unstimulated eosinophils to PCG or HMVEC was observed, suggesting that resting cells may adhere via alternative, perhaps non-specific, mechanisms. Although larger numbers of eosinophils were observed to adhere to PCG, comparable results were given in both adherence assays in terms of the percentage increase compared with baseline adherence. These observations confirm that

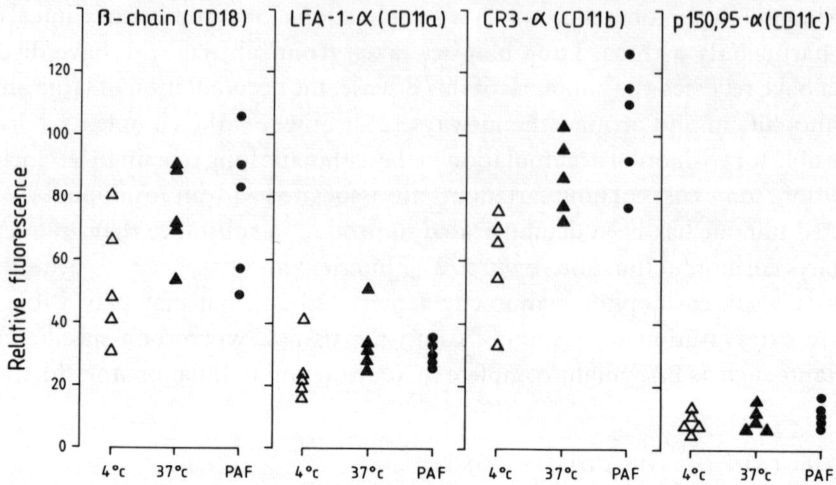

Fig. 6.5. Analysis of resting and PAF (10^{-6} M) -stimulated eosinophil CD11/18 expression using monoclonal antibodies and flow cytometry.

eosinophil hyperadhesion *in vitro* to PCG and HMVEC is a specific event, requiring the presence of specific membrane molecules and that enhanced adhesion appears dependent upon a change in receptor affinity or confirmation.

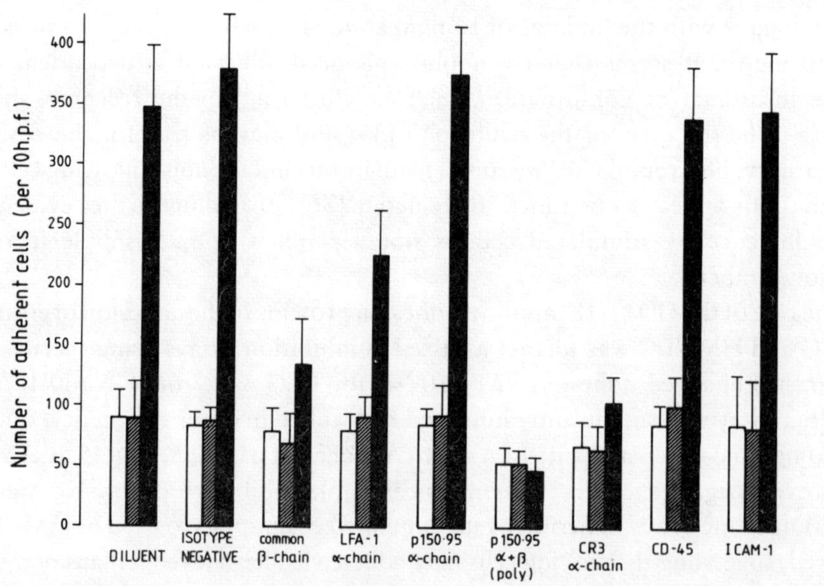

Fig. 6.6 Inhibition of resting and PAF (10^{-6} M) -stimulated eosinophil adherence to PCG by specific monoclonal antibodies to the CD11/18 adhesion proteins. Each point represents the mean ± SEM of five experiments. (□) Buffer, (▨) L-PAF (10^{-6} M), (■) PAF (10^{-6} M).

Conclusion

Our observations with PAF agree closely with the findings of Kimani *et al.* [15], in both dose–response and the kinetics of the response. These workers conducted their studies utilizing HVEC and serum coated plastic plates and also demonstrated inhibition of PAF-induced eosinophil hyperadherence (but not baseline adherence) by an anti-common β-chain mcAb. We have extended these observations to include the other members of the CD11/18 complex, i.e. LFA-1α, CR3α and p150, 95α. Anti-CR3 and common β-chain gave the greatest levels of inhibition, LFA-1 resulted in approximately 50% reduction in adherent cell numbers, with little effect given by p150,95. The large inhibitory effect of anti-β-chain may reflect intrinsic adhesive determinants on the β molecule. However, the possibility of secondary blockade by the β-subunit impairing the functional activities of the α-subunits cannot be excluded. Interestingly baseline adhesion by resting cells was not influenced by prior incubation with mcAbs, suggesting that unstimulated cells may adhere via other perhaps non-specific mechanisms. Our data are in broad agreement with published observations with regard to neutrophil adherence and its inhibition by anti-CD11/18 mcAbs [37,38], which appear to utilize CR3 and to a lesser extent LFA-1 in adherence reactions. CR3 is known to bind to HUVEC, plastic and PCG via a 'lectin-like' site, which is distinct from its passive C3bi binding site [37,38]. However, the adhesive ligand on endothelial cells has yet to be identified, as is the moiety on PCG or plastic by which

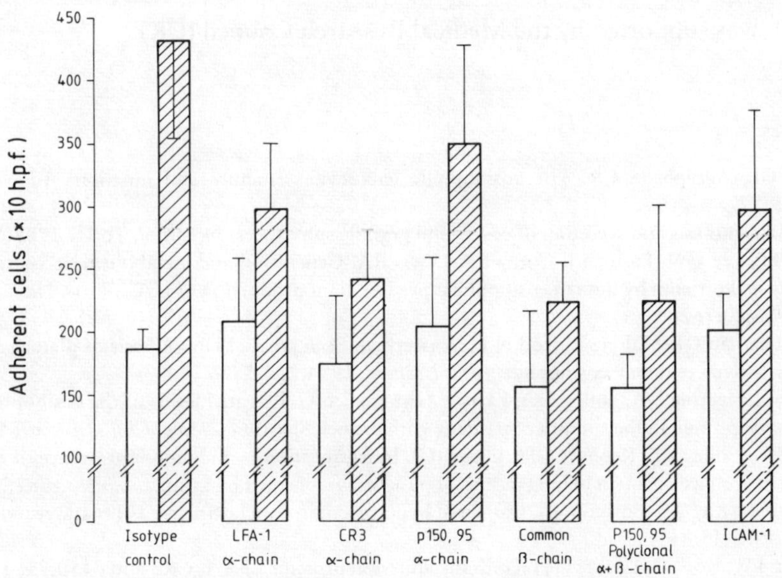

Fig. 6.7. Inhibition of resting and IL-5 (60 IU/ml) -stimulated eosinophil adherence to cultured HMVEC by monoclonal antibodies against the CD11/18 adhesion complex. Each point represents the mean ± SEM of four experiments. (□) Diluent, (▨) IL-5 (120 IU/ml).

eosinophils and other phagocytic cells bind. Given the close similarity between eosinophil and neutrophil expression of CD11/18 membrane adhesion proteins [13], the similarities between eosinophil and neutrophil adhesion reactions, are perhaps not surprising. Furthermore, it must be remembered that endothelial cells possess distinct adhesion receptors, including ICAM-1 and endothelial–leucocyte adhesion molecule (ELAM) and that these are amenable to upregulation following cell activation [10–12]. Lamas *et al.* [39] have demonstrated that incubation of HVEC, derived from human umbilical cord, with cytokines such as IL-1 and TNF results in increased adherence *in vitro* by unstimulated human eosinophils, most likely as a result of upregulation of ICAM and/or ELAM. Finally the possibility of the eosinophil possessing adhesion receptors distinct from the CD11/18 family cannot be excluded.

In conclusion, there is now a growing body of data suggesting that *in vitro* eosinophil hyperadherence is similar to that of the neutrophil, requiring the presence of specific adhesion proteins of the CD11/18 receptor complex. However enhanced adhesion appears dependent upon an affinity or confirmational change in the receptor(s) and not increased expression. The observation that IL-5 is a selective enhancer of eosinophil adherence to PCG and HMVEC may provide some insight into the preferential eosinophil accumulation observed in allergic-type inflammation, particularly asthma.

Acknowledgement

This work was supported by the Medical Research Council (UK).

References

1 Gleich GL, Adolphson CR. The eosinophilic leukocyte: structure and function. *Adv. Immunol.* 1986;**39**:177.

2 Spry CJF. Synthesis and secretion of eosinophil granule substances. *Immunol. Today* 1985;**6**:332.

3 Weller PF, Lee CW, Foster EJ, Corey KF, Lewis RA. Generation and metabolism of 5-lipoxygenase pathway leukotrienes by human eosinophils: predominant production of LTC_4. *Proc. Natl. Acad. Sci. USA* 1983;**80**:7626.

4 Lee T, Lenihan DJ, Malone B, Roddy L, Wasserman SI. Increased biosynthesis of platelet activating factor in activated human eosinophils. *J. Biol. Chem.* 1984;**259**:5526.

5 Frigas E, Loegering DA, Solley GO, Farrow GM, Gleich G. Elevated levels of the eosinophil granule major basic protein in the sputum of patients with bronchial asthma. *Mayo Clin. Proc.* 1981;**56**:345.

6 Filley WV, Holley KE, Kephart GM, Gleich GJ. Indentification by immunofluorescence of eosinophil granule major basic protein in lung tissues of patients with bronchial asthma. *Lancet* 1982;**ii**:11.

7 Durham SR, Kay AB. Eosinophils, bronchial hyperreactivity and late phase asthmatic reactions. *Clin. Allergy* 1985;**15**:411.

8 Kuypers TW, Roos D. Leukocyte membrane adhesion proteins LFA-1, CR3 and p150,95: a review of functional and regulatory aspects. *Res. Immunol.* 1989;**140**:461.

9 Anderson DC, Springer TA. Leukocyte adhesion deficiency: an inherited defect in the Mac-1, LFA-1 and p150,95 glycoproteins. *Ann. Rev. Med.* 1987;**38**:175.

10 Dustin ML, Rothlein R, Bhan AK, Dinarello CA. Springer TA. Induction by IL-1 and interferon-gamma: tissue distribution, biochemistry and function of natural adherence molecule (ICAM-1). *J. Immunol.* 1986;**137**:245.

11 Pohlman TH, Stanness KA, Beatty PG, Ochs HD, Harlan JM. An endothelial cell surface factor(s) induced *in vitro* by lipopolysaccharide, IL-1 and tumour necrosis factor-α increases neutrophil adherence by a CD18-dependent mechanism. *J. Immunol.* 1986;**136**:4538.

12 Bevilacqua MP, Pober JS, Mendrick DL, Cotran RS, Gimbrone MA. Identification of an inducable endothelial-leukocyte adhesion molecule. *Proc. Nat. Acad. Sci. USA* 1987;**84**:9238.

13 Hartnell A, Moqbel R, Walsh GM, Bradley B, Kay AB. Fcγ and CD11/18 receptor expression on normal density and low density human eosinophils. *Immunology* 1990;**69**:264–270.

14 Wardlaw AJ, Moqbel R, Cromwell O, Kay AB. PAF-acether is a chemotactic and chemokinetic factor for human eosinophils. *J. Clin. Invest.* 1986;**78**:1701.

15 Kimani G, Tonnesen MG, Henson PM. Stimulation of eosinophil adherence to human vascular endothelial cells *in vitro* by platelet activating factor. *J. Immunol.* 1988;**140**:3161.

16 MacDonald AJ, Moqbel R, Wardlaw AJ, Kay AB. Platelet activating factor (PAF) enhances eosinophil cytotoxicity *in vitro*. *J. Allergy Clin. Immunol.* 1986;**77**:227 (abstract no. 427).

17 Walsh GM, Moqbel R, Wardlaw AJ, Kay AB. *In vitro* effects of chemotactic factors on eosinophil Fc and complement receptor expression. *Acta Paed. Jpn.* 1987;**29**:672.

18 Bussolino F, Cammusi G, Aglietta M, Braquet P, Bosia A, Pescarmona G, Ganavio F, D'Urso N, Marchiso PC. Human endothelial cells are target for platelet activating factor. *J. Immunol.* 1987;**139**:2439.

19 Owen WF, Rothenberg ME, Silberstein DS, Gasson JC, Stevens RL, Austin KF, Soberman RJ. Regulation of human eosinophil viability, density and function by granulocyte/macrophage colony-stimulating factor in the presence of 3t3 fibroblasts. *J. Exp. Med.* 1987;**166**:129.

20 Rothenberg ME, Owen WF, Silberstein DS, Woods J, Soberman RJ, Austin KF, Stevens RL. Human eosinophils have prolonged survival, enhanced functional properties and become hypodense when exposed to human interleukin-3. *J. Clin. Invest.* 1988;**81**:1986.

21 Saito H, Hatake K, Dvorak AM, Leiferman KM, Donnenberg AD, Arai N, Ishizaka K, Ishizaka T. Selective differentiation and proliferation of haematopoietic cells induced by recombinant human interleukins. *Proc. Natl. Acad. Sci. USA* 1988;**85**:2288.

22 Lopez AF, Sanderson CJ, Gamble JR, Campbell HR, Young IG, Vadas MA. Recombinant human interleukin-5 is a selective activator of human eosinophil function. *J. Exp. Med.* 1988;**167**:225.

23 Yamaguchi Y, Hayashi Y, Sugama Y, Miura Y, Kasahara T, Kitamura S, Torisu M, Mita S, Tominaga A, Takatsu K, Suda T. Highly purified murine interleukin 5 (IL-5) stimulates eosinophil function and prolongs *in vitro* survival. *J. Exp. Med.* 1988;**176**:1737.

24 Vadas MA, David JR, Butterworth AE, Pisani NT, Siongok TA. A new method for the purification of human eosinophils and neutrophils and a comparison of the ability of these cells to damage schistosomula of *Schistosoma mansoni*. *J. Immunol.* 1979;**122**:1228.

25 Dunnill MS, Masseralla GR, Anderson JA. A comparison of the quantitative anatomy of the bronchi in normal subjects, in status asthmaticus, in chronic bronchitis and in emphysema. *Thorax* 1969;**24**:176.

26 Spry CJF, Weetman AP, Olsson I, Tai P–C, Olsen EG. The pathogenesis of eosinophilic endomyocardial disease in patients with carcinomas of the lung. *Heart Vessels* 1985;**1**:162.

27 Kodama T, Takada K, Kaymeya Y, Shimosato R, Tsuchiya R, Okabe T. Large cell carcinoma of the lung associated with marked eosinophilia. *Cancer (Phila.)* 1984;**54**:2313.

28 Numao T, Fukuda T, Akutsu I, Makino S, Enokihara H, Honjo T. Selective enhancement of eosinophil chemotaxis by recombinant human interleukin-5 *J. Allergy Clin. Immunol.* 1989;**83**:298 (abstract no. 508).

29 Aranout MA, Colten HR. Complement C3 receptors: structure and function. *Mol. Immunol.* 1984;**21**:1191.

30 Berger M, O'Shea J, Cross AS, Folks TM, Chused TM, Brown EJ, Frank MM. Human neutrophils increase expression of C3bi as well as C3b receptors upon activation. *J. Clin. Invest.* 1984;**74**:1566.

31 Springer TA, Miller LF, Anderson DC. p150,95, the third member of the MAC-1, LFA-1, human leukocyte adhesion glycoprotein family. *J. Immunol.* 1986;**136**:240.

32 Shalit M, von Allmen C, Atkins PC, Zweiman B. Platelet activating factor increases expression of complement receptors on human neutrophils. *J. Leuk. Biol.* 1988;**44**:212.

33 Vedder NB, Harlan JM. Increased surface expression of CD11b/CD18 (Mac-1) is not required for stimulated neutrophil adherence to cultured endothelium. *J. Clin. Invest.*1988;**81**:676.

34 Phillips MR, Buyon JP, Winchester R, Weissmann G, Abramson SB. Upregulation of the iC3b receptor (CR3) is neither necessary nor sufficient to promote neutrophil aggregation. *J. Clin. Invest.* 1988;**82**:495.

35 Detmers PA, Wright SD, Olsen E, Kimball B, Cohn ZA. Aggregation of complement receptors on human neutrophils in the absence of ligand. *J. Cell Biol.* 1988;**105**:1137.

36 Buyon JP, Abramson SB, Phillips MR, Slade SG, Ross GD, Weissmann G, Winchester RJ. Dissociation between increased surface expression of gp165/95 and homotypic neutrophil aggregation.*J. Immunol.* 1988;**140**:3156.

37 Anderson DC, Miller LJ, Schmalsteig FC, Rothlein R, Springer TA. Contributions of the MAC-1 glycoprotein family to adherence-dependent granulocytic functions: structure–function assessments employing subunit-specific monoclonal antibodies. *J. Immunol.* 1986;**137**:15.

38 Wallis WJ, Hickstein DD, Schwartz BR, June CH, Ochs HD, Beatty PG, Klebanoff SJ, Harlan JM. Monoclonal antibody-defined functional epitopes on the adhesion-promoting glycoprotein complex (CD18) of human neutrophils. *Blood* 1986;**67**:1007.

39 Lamas AM, Mulroney CM, Schleimer RP. Studies of the adhesive interaction between purified human eosinophils and cultured vascular endothelial cells. *J. Immunol.* 1988;**140**:1500.

7 · IgE-dependent eosinophil effector mechanisms

R. Moqbel,* A.J. MacDonald, G.M. Walsh and A.B. Kay

Summary

Using human IgE and a number of *in vitro* assays, i.e. the rosette technique, flow cytometry, cytotoxicity and mediator (leukotriene C_4) release, we have shown that low density eosinophils were involved in IgE-dependent effector functions. Normal density eosinophils, on the other hand, did not respond in IgE-dependent systems, but putative receptors for IgE appeared to be amenable to upregulation by pretreatment with allergic mediators. Platelet-activating factor (PAF) was most potent in influencing these IgE-dependent reactions compared with leukotriene (LT) B_4 and histamine. These results suggest that eosinophils, which are important elements of IgE-dependent hypersensitivity, may participate in IgE-dependent effector function(s) in allergic disorders.

Introduction

Allergic inflammation and immunity to a number of tissue dwelling helminthic infections, are associated with elevations in total and allergen-specific IgE and increases in the number of peripheral and tissue eosinophils. Eosinophils possess a number of membrane receptors including those for complement components C3b and iC3b (CR1 and CR3) [1] and the receptor for IgG (FcγRII) [2]. These receptors are thought to be involved in the process of cell adherence, mediator release and *in vitro* cytotoxicity against appropriately opsonized helminthic targets [3–5]. *In vitro* activation of eosinophils by chemotactic factors results in enhanced expression of these receptors and seems to be associated with increases in their effector function [6–8].

Low density (hypodense) eosinophils obtained from patients with hypereosinophilia (e.g. hypereosinophilic syndrome) appear to be metabolically more 'activated' than normal density (normodense) eosinophils, obtained from mild eosinophilic subjects [9]. It has been suggested that these cells exhibit a higher expression of receptors for IgE, which has been designated as FcεRII [10]. This receptor was described in both rat and human eosinophils [11] and shown to consist of two polypeptide chains of 50 and 25 kD [12] with a low (1.17×10^{-7} mol/l) binding affinity [13]. IgE receptors (FcεRII) on B-cells (CD23) and other inflammatory cells (e.g. platelets and macrophages) have also been described, but their relationship with 'similar' receptors

*To whom correspondence should be addressed.

on eosinophils remains unclear. However, two distinct forms of FcεRII have been described recently: FcεRIIa present only on B-cells and FcεRIIb which appears to be expressed on a number of inflammatory cells, including eosinophil cell lines [14].

An essential element in the study of the role of IgE in relation to normal and hypodense eosinophils is the use of purified IgE. This was achieved using either myeloma IgE protein or purified antigen-specific IgE fractions from immune serum using a combination of fast protein liquid chromatography (FPLC) and affinity chromatography. Using these purified proteins we have also investigated the effect of the potent eosinophilotactic agent [15], PAF, and other allergic mediators on eosinophil IgE-dependent functions.

IgE receptor expression on human eosinophils

Rosettes

Normal density eosinophils were treated by PAF, its biologically inactive precursor and metabolite, lyso-PAF, LTB_4, histamine and the synthetic tripeptide formyl-methionyl-leucyl-phenylalanine (FMLP) prior to use in an IgE-dependent rosette assay employing sheep erythrocytes coated with human myeloma IgE protein. Platelet-activating factor and LTB_4, but not lyso-PAF, were equipotent in inducing

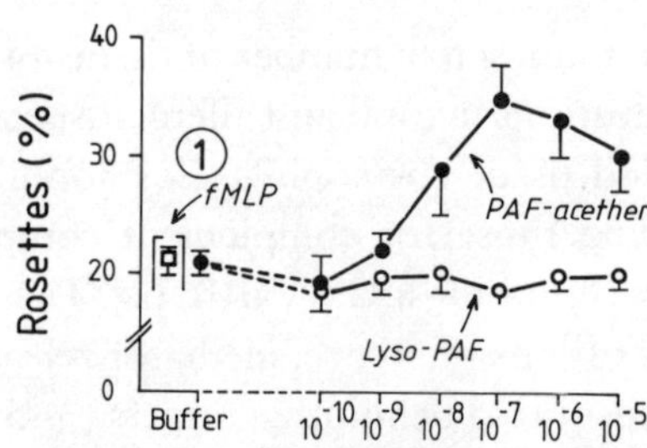

Fig. 7.1. The effect of PAF, lyso-PAF, LTB_4 and histamine on IgE rosettes on normal density eosinophils. Formyl-methionyl-leucyl-phenylalanine was used at a single concentration of 10^{-7} mol/l ($n = 4$).

significant ($p < 0.01$) dose-dependent increases in percentage IgE rosettes (optimal at 10^{-7} mol/l). A period of 30 min with the optimal dose of each of these autacoids was required to effect maximum enhancement. Histamine enhanced IgE-dependent rosettes but to a lesser extent than PAF and LTB_4 ($p < 0.05$) and at a higher molar concentration (10^{-5} mol/l). In contrast, FMLP did not enhance IgE rosettes (Fig. 7.1).

Flow cytometry

The above IgE-dependent effector mechanisms were further studied using flow cytometry, a fluorescein-conjugated polyclonal anti-IgE antibody and native human myeloma IgE protein to examine the ability of normal density eosinophils to bind IgE. Unstimulated cells in the absence of added IgE protein exhibited measurable fluorescence suggesting that 15% of that cell population bear cytophilic IgE on their surface. When the cells were preincubated with myeloma IgE at 4°C before adding the IgE-FITC conjugated antibody, the fluorescence only increased slightly, indicative of the occupation of most available receptors by IgE protein acquired *in vivo*. However, when these cells were preincubated with PAF, LTB_4 or histamine but not lyso-PAF or FMLP, the uptake of greater quantities of native IgE by these stimulated cells was observed as expressed by enhanced fluorescence (up to 100% in the case of PAF) (Fig. 7.2). Platelet-activating factor gave a time- and dose-dependent increase in IgE binding (optimal at 10^{-7} mol/l). Leukotriene B_4 gave a smaller but significant ($p < 0.01$) increase in IgE binding compared with PAF, but only at 10^{-7} mol/l, while histamine

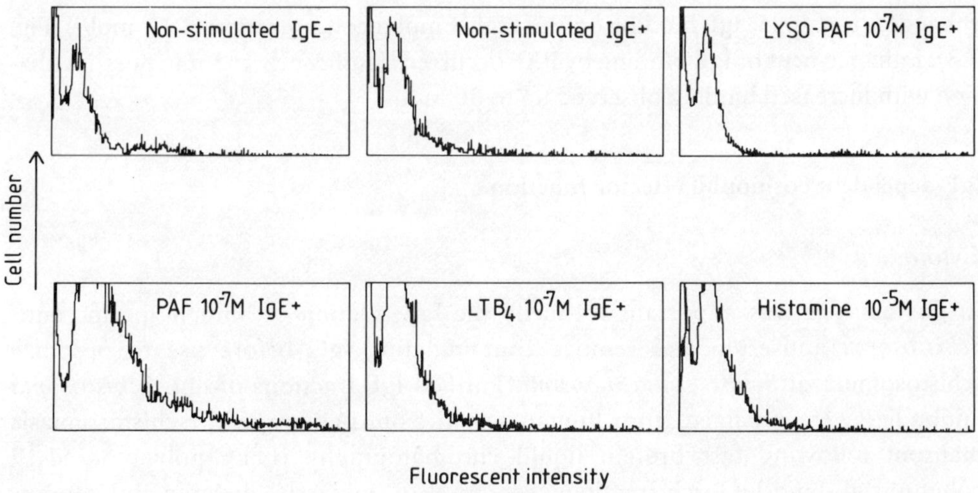

Fig. 7.2. A representative tracing of an experiment showing flow cytometric analysis of normal cytophilic IgE levels, uptake of native IgE by resting eosinophils and increased uptake following stimulation by chemotactic factors.

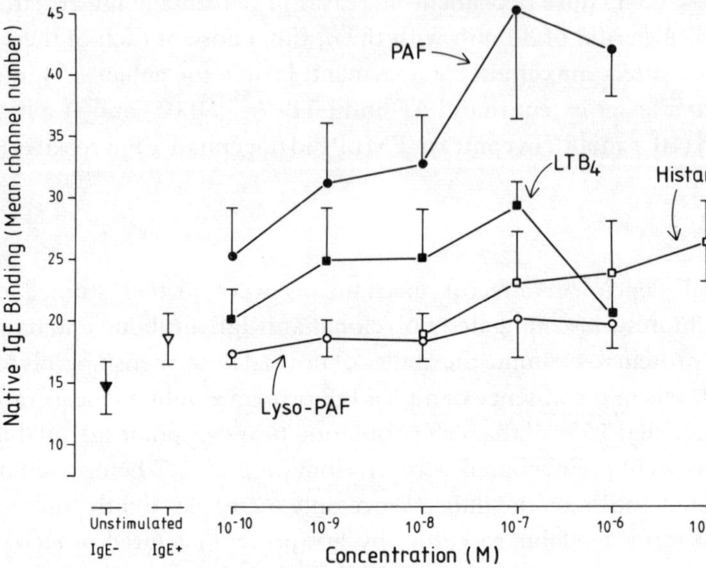

Fig. 7.3. A comparison of enhanced eosinophil IgE binding by chemotactic mediators. Purified normal human eosinophils were incubated with increasing concentrations of PAF, lyso-PAF, LTB_4, histamine or RPMI+ for 30 min at 37°C. Following incubation with native IgE and an FITC-conjugated anti-IgE, the cells were analysed for fluorescence on the basis of their light scattering properties. Cytophilic IgE levels were also measured. Results are expressed as mean channel fluorescence, with the negative binding control readings subtracted ($n = 5$).

enhanced ($p < 0.05$) IgE binding only at higher molar concentration (10^{-5} mol/l) (Fig. 7.3). Enhancement of IgE binding by PAF occurred significantly at 5 min post-incubation with increased binding observed up to 30 min.

IgE-dependent eosinophil effector function

Cytotoxicity

In this assay it was important to purify the IgE fraction of human specific anti-*Schistosoma* antiserum and remove contaminating IgG before use to opsonize schistosomula of *Schistosoma mansoni.* Purified IgE fractions of anti-*Schistosoma* antibodies were obtained from human serum from patients with schistosomiasis mansoni following fast protein liquid chromatography (FPLC-polyanion SI-17 column). IgE- and IgG-rich fractions were pooled separately, dialysed and concentrated. *Schistosoma mansoni*-specific IgE and IgG were identified and their amounts measured by modified RAST and ELISA assays, respectively. IgG contaminating the IgE-rich fractions was removed by adsorption on a *Staphylococcus aureus*–protein A affinity column, without influencing the levels of IgE. Schistosomula were coated (2 h, 20°C) with purified IgE fractions, before and after protein A and anti-IgE affinity columns and then incubated with eosinophils in the *in vitro* cytotoxocity assay [4]. Percentage of killed larvae was determined 24 h later by a visual assay.

Table 7.1. IgG- and IgE-rich fractions of immune anti-*Schistosoma* serum. Effects of various adsorption manoeuvres on levels of specific IgG and IgE and their ability, when used to coat live and fixed schistosomula, to elicit hypodense eosinophil cytotoxicity and LTC_4 release, respectively

	Specific anti-*Schistosoma* IgE and IgG		Hypodense eosinophils	
Opsonin	IgE % binding (RAST)	IgG units (OD) (ELISA)	Cytotoxicity (% kill)	LTC_4 release (pmol/10^6 cells)
Unfractionated immune serum	36	8.4	82±5	15±4
IgE-rich fractions, untreated	35	7.0	31±1	7.8±0.4
IgE-rich fractions+protein A adsorption	32	0.18	30±1.5	5.5±0.4
IgE-rich fractions + anti-IgE adsorption	0	6.4	11±2	0.25±0.1
IgE-rich fractions + protein A + anti-IgE adsorption	0	0.2	8±3	0.2±0.2
IgG-rich fractions, untreated	0	6.8	40±2	6.0±0.1
IgG-rich fractions + protein A adsorption	0	0.1	9.4±4	0.1±0.1
IgG-rich fractions + anti-IgE adsorption	0	6.0	35±3	5.6±0.3

Human hypodense eosinophils mediated the killing of IgE-coated schistosomula in the absence of any IgG contamination. This effect was confirmed by showing that the IgE-dependent response was ablated by adsorption of IgE onto an anti-IgE-affinity column (Table 7.1). In contrast, normodense eosinophils exhibited negligible ability to kill IgE-coated schistosomula but their cytotoxic capacity was enhanced following their stimulation with PAF (optimal at 10^{-8} mol/l), LTB_4 (optimal at 10^{-7} mol/l) and histamine (optimal at 10^{-5} mol/l), but not lyso-PAF or FMLP. The latter, however, was able to enhance IgG-dependent killing (optimal enhancement at 10^{-7} mol/l).

IgE-dependent mediator release

The above study was extended to examine the ability of eosinophils to release their major membrane phospholipid-derived and lipoxygenase metabolite, LTC_4, in IgE-dependent systems. For this purpose, both live and killed (formalin-fixed) schistosomula were used. These were coated with anti-*Schistosoma* serum (containing

Table 7.2. Eosinophil-derived LTC_4 release following stimulation with opsonized schistosomula, IgG-coated beads or calcium ionophore ($n = 7$)

Stimulus	Immunoreactive LTC_4 (pmol/10^6 cells)
Live schistosomula+immune serum	11.7±2.7
Fixed schistosomula+immune serum	16.5±3.5
Live schistosomula+diluent	0.1±0.1
Fixed schistosomula+diluent	0.1±0.1
IgG-coated beads	9.9±1
A23187 (5×10^{-6} M)	80.0±24
Untreated cells	0

specific IgE, IgG and complement). These opsonized schistosomula elicited the release of 11.7±2.7 and 16.5±3.5 pmol of $LTC_4/1\times10^6$ eosinophils from live and fixed larvae, respectively (Table 7.2). The amounts of LTC_4 elaborated by eosinophils following adherence to live and fixed schistosomula represented 14.7 and 20.6% of the total LTC_4 generated from these cells after calcium ionophore A23187 treatment (5×10^{-6} mol/l); they were also comparable with amounts elaborated in the presence of the physiological trigger [16] in the presence of Sepharose beads covalently-coated with normal human IgG. When fixed schistosomula were coated with FPLC-purified IgE fractions (as described above) they elicited the release of 11.6±0.4 pmol of LTC_4 from 10^6 low density eosinophils (Table 7.1). This activity was also ablated by IgE adsorption in a similar fashion to that described for cytotoxicity. Normal density eosinophils, on the other hand, were unable to generate LTC_4 in the presence of schistosomula coated with a specific IgE-, but were able to do so in the presence of IgG-coated schistosomula. The IgE-dependent response was only effective in terms of

Table 7.3. The effect of a number of chemotactic factors on the release of LTC_4 from human eosinophils (both normal and low density) elicited by IgG- and IgE-coated schistosomula. Cells were preincubated with the mediators for 30 min prior to incubation with IgE-opsonized schistosomula for 45 min (37°C, 5% CO_2)

	Immunoreactive LTC_4 (pmol/10^6 eosinophils)			
	Normal density		Low density	
Treatment	IgG-rich	IgE-rich	IgG-rich	IgE-rich
Untreated	5.3	0.4	7.1	6.3
PAF 10^{-7} M	6.8	4.4	8.9	7.9
Lyso-PAF 10^{-7} M	4.0	0.6	6.2	5.8
LTB_4 10^{-7} M	6.5	3.6	7.2	6.9
FMLP 10^{-7} M	10.8	1.1	10.3	6.8

measurement of LTC_4 in the supernatant, when normodense eosinophils were preincubated with PAF or LTB_4 (both used at an optimal dose of 10^{-7} mol/l) (Table 7.3). Neither lyso-PAF nor FMLP had any influence on the ability of normal density eosinophils to elaborate LTC_4 in the presence of IgE-coated larvae.

Conclusion

Our results suggest that low-density eosinophils appear to be involved in IgE-dependent effector functions, as measured by the ability of eosinophils to be cytotoxic against, and release a major lipid mediator (LTC_4) following adherence to, larvae coated with purified parasite-specific IgE. These activities, that appeared to be absent in normal density eosinophils, were upregulated following activation by PAF, LTB_4 and to a lesser extent histamine. Such upregulation was confirmed by studies using flow cytometry, which demonstrated that stimulated eosinophils bound a myeloma IgE. Platelet-activating factor was also the most potent autacoid in this system and its ability to influence the binding of IgE on eosinophils was shown to be inhibitable by a specific PAF antagonist (SDZ 64–412) in a dose-dependent fashion [Walsh, Nagakura, Iikura, unpublished observations].

Chemotactic factor-induced enhancement of IgE-dependent effector function may be related to the ability of these mediators to influence membrane events by either increasing surface receptor numbers or effecting a conformational change in these receptors. Platelet-activating factor and to a lesser extent LTB_4, seem to be potent in influencing IgE-dependent activities of normal eosinophils. This may have important implications within the context of allergic hypersensitivity disorders where these responses are known to be deleterious. On the other hand, similar IgE-dependent, eosinophil-mediated functions may contribute 'beneficially' towards protective inflammatory mechanisms within the mucosal tissues of sensitized mammalian hosts as a response to re-invading worm infections.

Acknowledgements

This work was supported by the Medical Research Council and Sandoz (Japan) Ltd.

References

1 Fischer E, Capron M, Prin L, Kusnierz JP, Kazatchkine MD. Human eosinophils express CR1 and CR3 complement receptors for cleavage fragments of C3. *Cell Immunol.* 1986;97:297.

2 Kulczycki A, Jr. Human neutrophils and eosinophils have structurally distinct Fc receptors. *J. Immunol.* 1984;133:849.

3 Kimani G, Tonnesen MG, Henson PM. Stimulation of eosinophil adherence to human vascular endothelial cells *in vitro* by platelet-activating factor. *J. Immunol.* 1988;140:3161.

4 Spry CJF. Synthesis and secretion of eosinophil granule substances. *Immunol. Today* 1985;6:332.

5 Butterworth AE. Cell-mediated damage to helminths. *Adv. Parasitol.* 1984;23:143.

6 Anwar ARE, McKean JR, Smithers SR, Kay AB. Human eosinophil- and neutrophil-mediated killing of schistosomula of *Schistosoma mansoni in vitro*. I. Enhancement of complement-dependent damage by mast cell-derived mediators and formyl-methionyl peptides. *J. Immunol.* 1980;**124**:1122.

7 Nagy L, Lee TH, Goetzl EJ, Pickett WC, Kay AB. Complement receptor enhancement and chemotaxis of human neutrophils and eosinophils by leukotrienes and other lipoxygenase products. *Clin. Exp. Immunol.* 1982;**47**:541.

8 Moqbel R, Sass-Kuhn SP, Goetzl EJ, Kay AB. Enhancement of neutrophil- and eosinophil-mediated complement-dependent killing of schistosomula of *Schistosoma mansoni, in vitro,* by leukotriene B_4. *Clin. Exp. Immunol.* 1983;**52**:519.

9 Prin L, Capron M, Tonnel AB, Bletry O, Capron A. Heterogeneity of human eosinophils; variability in cell density and cytotoxic ability in relation to the level and the origin of hypereosinophilia. *Int. Arch. Allergy. Appl. Immunol.* 1983;**72**:336.

10 Capron M, Capron A. The IgE receptor of human eosinophils. In *Allergy and Inflammation,* (Ed. Kay AB). Academic Press, London, p. 151.

11 Capron M, Capron A, Dessaint JP, Torpier G, Johansson SGO, Prin L. Fc receptors for IgE on human and rat eosinophils. *J. Immunol.* 1981;**126**:2087.

12 Capron M, Kusnierz JP, Prin L, Spiegelberg HL, Ovlague G, Gosset Ph, Tonnel AB, Capron A. Cytophilic IgE on human blood and tissue eosinophils: detection by flow microfluorometry. *J. Immunol.* 1985;**134**:3013.

13 Jouault T, Capron M, Balloul JM, Ameisen JC, Capron A. Quantitative and qualitative analysis of the Fc receptor for IgE (FcεRII) on human eosinophils. *Eur. J. Immunol.* 1988;**18**:237.

14 Yokota A, Kikutano H, Tanaka T, Sato R, Barsumian EL, Suemura M, Kishimoto T. Two species of human Fc-epsilon receptor II (FcεRII/CD23): tissue-species and IL-4-specific regulation of gene expression. *Cell* 1988;**55**:611.

15 Wardlaw AJ, Moqbel R, Cromwell O, Kay AB. Platelet activating factor. A potent chemotactic and chemokinetic factor for human eosinophils. *J. Clin. Invest.* 1986;**78**:1701.

16 Shaw RJ, Walsh GM, Cromwell O, Moqbel R, Spry CJF, Kay AB. Activated human eosinophils generate SRS-A leukotrienes after physiological (IgG-dependent) stimulation. *Nature* 1985;**316**:150.

8 · Eosinophils and pulmonary hyperresponsiveness in the rat

R.C. Baker, R.M. Cook, Pat A. Hatt, Sarah M. Laycock, N.R.J. Musgrove, H. Smith* and Barbara A. Spicer

Summary

Rats given Sephadex particles intravenously had a blood and tissue eosinophilia and a pulmonary hyperresponsiveness to 5-hydroxytryptamine (5-HT). The hyperresponsiveness was shown as a hypersensitivity to the respiratory effects of 5-HT *in vivo,* with a parallel shift to the left of the intravenous dose–response curve. *In vitro* lung strips from Sephadex treated rats were hyperreactive; they responded over the same dose range of 5-HT as strips from control rats but the slope of the dose–response curve was greater. There was a correlation between the number of blood eosinophils and the pulmonary hypersensitivity *in vivo* and hyperreactivity *in vitro*. Peritoneal eosinophils collected from Sephadex treated rats showed enhanced chemiluminescent and cytotoxicity responses.

Introduction

Asthma is characterized by a pulmonary airways hyperresponsiveness, to a variety of stimuli, and an eosinophilia. The number of blood eosinophils correlates with the severity of the disease [1] and the airways responsiveness to inhaled histamine [2]. Many attempts have been made to produce models of airways hyperresponsiveness in animals by allowing them to inhale noxious substances which have ranged from antigen to nitric acid. The increase in responsiveness of the airways of the animals to subsequent challenge with a spasmogen could be produced by a variety of mechanisms, for example: an increase in vascular permeability would increase the amount of spasmogen absorbed and distributed to the pulmonary smooth-muscle; extravasation of plasma proteins and damage to the bronchial epithelium might prime nerve receptors, and; the nature of the pulmonary smooth-muscle might be changed, in which case this should be shown as a change in responsiveness of the pulmonary tissue *in vitro*.

We have used a different approach. We have produced an eosinophilia in the rat and determined the effect of this on the responsiveness of pulmonary tissue *in vivo* and *in vitro*. We chose the rat in preference to the guinea pig since normal guinea pigs in

*To whom correspondence should be addressed.

comparison with most other animals investigated, including normal man, have a relatively high proportion of eosinophils in their bronchoalveolar lavage (BAL) fluids [3].

A blood eosinophilia can be produced in rats by the intravenous injection of Sephadex or protein coated latex particles of the appropriate size to embolize in the vasculature [4 for references]. It is possible that the particles mimic the blood migratory phase of some helminth parasites. In the current study we used Sephadex particles.

Materials and methods

These were as described [4–6], briefly.

Animals. Male Charles River Sprague–Dawley rats, 250–350 g, were used.

Dosing. Sephadex G-200 was suspended in saline and 1 ml of the suspension was injected intravenously.

Eosinophil numbers were counted in: (a) blood from the tail vein; (b) bronchoalveolar lavage (BAL) fluids. Pooled washings from each rat were centrifuged and the cell pellet was suspended in 0.5 ml of saline. Numbers of leucocytes were quoted as millions/ml in this 0.5 ml; (c) lung tissue.

Airways responsiveness to 5-HT was measured: in vivo by the resistance to artificial respiration [4]; *in vitro* in lung strips under isometric tension [5].

Collection of peritoneal eosinophils. Saline, (5 ml) was injected intraperitoneally into rats and peritoneal washings were collected after 48 h. The eosinophils were purified to > 90% using discontinuous gradients of metrizamide.

Results

A single intravenous injection of Sephadex G-200 particles, 0.5 mg/rat in 1 ml of saline produced an increase in numbers of eosinophils in the blood peaking 7 days later and returning to control levels by day 14. A second injection of Sephadex given on day 14 produced an increase in numbers of eosinophils in the blood greater than the first peaking on day 19 and returning to control levels by day 25. The numbers of eosinophils in the blood, as millions/ml (mean ± SEM, $n = 9$ or more), were 0.17±0.07 on day 0 before giving the Sephadex, 0.32±0.23 ($p < 0.001$) on day 7, and 0.67±0.06 ($p < 0.001$) on day 19. Sephadex particles given to the rats on day 0 and 14 produced a dose-dependent increase in numbers of eosinophils in the blood, BAL fluids and lung tissue on day 19 (Fig. 8.1). There was no increase in numbers of

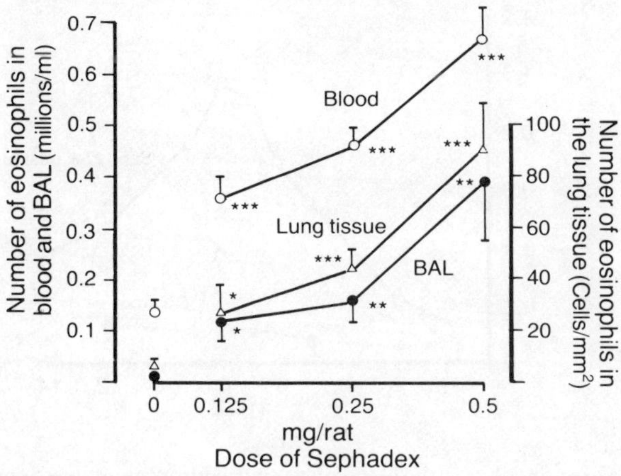

Fig. 8.1. The effects of injecting Sephadex, G-200, intravenously into rats on days 0 and 14 on the number of eosinophils in the blood (○), BAL fluid (●), and lung tissue (△) on day 19. Mean values ± SEM, $n = 5$ or more, $^{*}p < 0.05$, $^{**}p < 0.01$, $^{***}p < 0.001$.

other leucocytes in the blood and BAL fluids. 5-Hydroxytryptamine injected intravenously into the rats produced a dose-dependent increase in resistance to respiratory airflow in the lung. Rats injected with Sephadex on days 0 and 14 showed an increase in sensitivity to the respiratory effects of 5-HT on day 19, which was dependent upon the dose of Sephadex, as shown by parallel shifts to the left of the 5-HT dose – response curve (Fig. 8.2). Rats given Sephadex, G-200, 0.5 mg in 1 ml of saline, by a

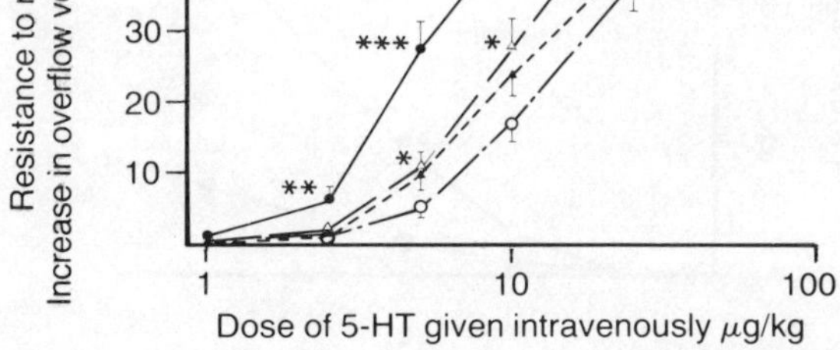

Fig. 8.2. Sensitivity of rats to the respiratory effects of 5-HT on day 19 after the intravenous injection of Sephadex particles, G-200, on days 0 and 14 at doses of, mg/rat; 0.5 (●); 0.25 (△) and 0.125 (▲), compared with rats given saline (○). The values are mean ± SEM for 12 animals, 2 dose – responses for each. $^{*}p = 0.05–0.01$; $^{**}p$ 0.01–0.001; $^{***}p < 0.001$.

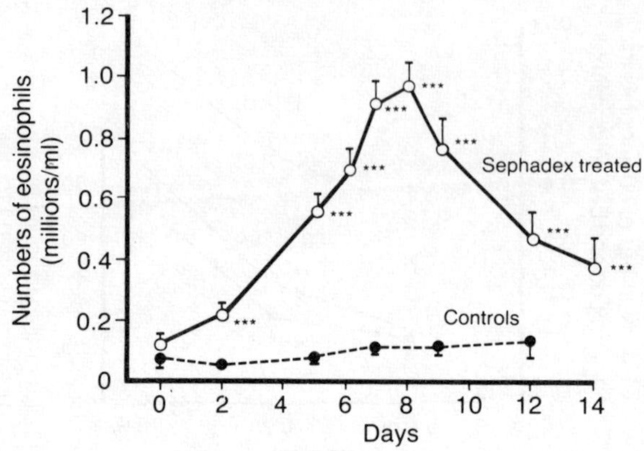

Fig. 8.3. The numbers of eosinophils in the blood of rats given intravenous injections of Sephadex, G-200, 0.5 mg in 1 ml of saline (○) or saline (●) on days 0, 2 and 5. Blood was collected before the injections on the days when they were given. The values are means ± SEM, $n = 6$ or more. $^{***}p < 0.001$ compared with mean value of controls. There were no changes in the numbers of other leucocytes in the blood at these times.

shortened dosage regimen, on days 0, 2 and 5 had an increase in numbers of eosinophils in their blood peaking on day 7 (Fig. 8.3) with no change in numbers of other leucocytes. In the BAL fluids of the rats on day 7 there was an increase in numbers of eosinophils, a decrease in numbers of mononuclear cells and a small increase in numbers of neutrophils. The values in millions/ml (mean ± SEM, $n = 24$ or more) were: control rats given saline, mononuclear cells 2.27±0.14, neutrophils

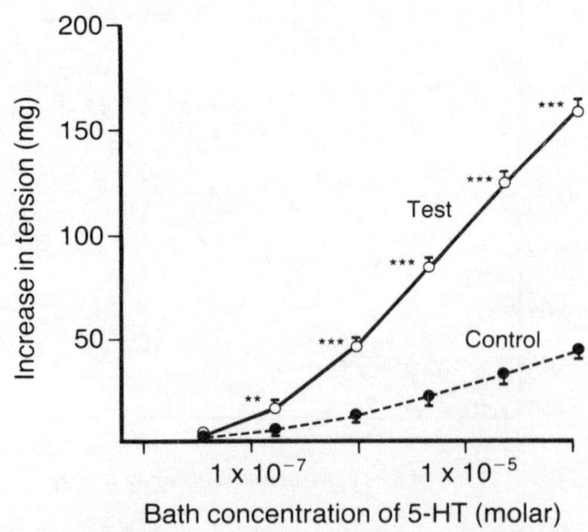

Fig. 8.4. The effect of 5-HT on lung parenchymal lung strips taken from rats dosed with Sephadex G-200, 0.5 mg, on days 0, 2 and 5. Strips were taken on days 6, 7, 8. Mean ± SEM, $n = 10$ or more. $^{**}p < 0.01$, $^{***}p < 0.001$.

0.05±0.006, eosinophils 0.02±0.02; for rats given Sephadex, mononuclear cells 1.36±0.06, $p < 0.001$, neutrophils 0.13±0.01, $p < 0.001$, eosinophils 0.68±0.04, $p < 0.001$. In the lungs, granuloma surrounding the Sephadex particles were present consisting mainly of mononuclear cells. There was a marked increase in numbers of eosinophils in the lung interstitial tissue between the vasculature and the bronchi with few eosinophils present in the alveolar septum.

Rats given Sephadex on day 0, 2 and 5 showed an increase in sensitivity to the respiratory effects of intravenously given 5-HT on day 7 with a parallel shift to the left of the dose – response curve compared with control rats given saline instead of Sephadex (data not shown). The effects were similar to those seen in rats on day 19 dosed with Sephadex G-200, 0.5 mg on days 0 and 14 (Fig. 8.2). Lung strips taken from rats given Sephadex were hyperreactive to 5-HT *in vitro* in that the lung strips from Sephadex treated and control rats responded over the same dose range of 5-HT but the response of the strips from the treated rats was greater (Fig. 8.4). From these and other studies there was a positive correlation between the numbers of blood eosinophils and pulmonary hypersensitivity to 5-HT *in vivo*, $r = 0.88$, $p < 0.001$, and hyperreactivity *in vitro*, $r = 0.76$, $p < 0.001$, $n > 100$.

Peritoneal washings were collected from rats 48 h after the intraperitoneal injection of saline. The intravenous injection of Sephadex G-200 at 0.5 mg a rat on days 0, 2 and 5 prior to the intraperitoneal injection of saline on day 7 increased the number of eosinophils in the peritoneal washings, collected on day 9, fourfold in comparison with the levels in rats given saline alone. The proportion of eosinophils was increased twofold to 40% of the total cells. Eosinophils obtained from rats given Sephadex and saline or saline alone were morphologically similar. None of the eosinophils had the vacuolated appearance associated with 'hypodense' or activated cells. The eosinophils obtained by the two methods contained similar levels of the cytoplasmic enzyme lactate dehydrogenase and the granule associated enzyme eosinophil peroxidase. The extracellular release of peroxidase from purified cells stimulated with complement-coated sepharose particles was also similar for each treatment. In contrast to these

Table 8.1. Activities of peritoneal eosinophils from rats given multiple injections of Sephadex

Treatment	% rosettes IgG Ab coated sheep red blood cells	% cytotoxicity to human K562 cells in presence of: IgG Ab	PMA	Chemi-luminescence PMA
Multiple Sephadex	45±4*	>30%	>70%	138.8±13.3%*
Untreated or single Sephadex[1]	22±6	<20%	<47%[1]	100%[1]

Mean ± SEM n=5 or more * p<0.01

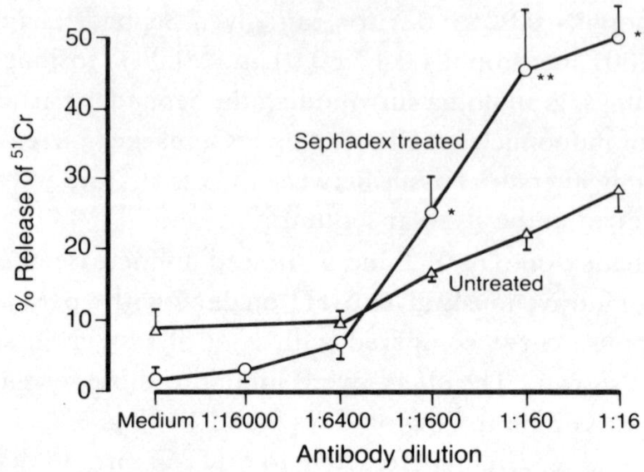

Fig. 8.5. Cytotoxicity to chicken erythrocytes of peritoneal eosinophils from rats given multiple doses of Sephadex or untreated, in the presence of Ab to the erythrocytes. Mean ± SEM, $n = 6$; $^{*}p < 0.05$; $^{**}p < 0.01$.

results eosinophils from animals given multiple injections of Sephadex showed an increased response to the soluble stimulus, phorbol myristate acetate (PMA), both in terms of oxidative metabolism and direct lysis of tumour target cells, and they also showed an increased activity in antibody-dependent assays (Table 8.1, Fig. 8.5).

In conclusion these results demonstrate that an induced eosinophilia in the rat can be associated with a pulmonary hyperresponsiveness, seen as hypersensitivity *in vivo*, and hyperreactivity of pulmonary tissue *in vitro*. A requirement could be that not only must eosinophils be present in sufficient numbers in the lung but they must also be activated.

References

1 Horn BR, Robin ED, Theodore J, van Kessel A. Total eosinophil counts in the management of asthma. *New Engl. J. Med.* 1975;**292**:1152–1155.

2 Taylor KJ, Luksza AR. Peripheral blood eosinophil counts and bronchial responsiveness. *Thorax* 1987;**42**:452–456.

3 Snella M–C, Venaille T, Holt P, Rylander R. Interstitial and free lung cells in acute inflammation in the guinea pig. *Agents Actions* 1987;**22**:261–269.

4 Laycock SM, Smith H, Spicer BA. Airway hyper-reactivity and blood, lung and airway eosinophilis in rats. *Int. Arch. Allergy Appl. Immun.* 1987;**81**:363–367.

5 Spicer BA, Baker R, Laycock SM, Smith H. Correlation between blood eosinophilia and airways hyperresponsiveness in rats. *Agents Actions* 1989;**26**:63–65.

6 Cook RM, Musgrove NRJ, Ashworth RF. Activity of rat peritoneal eosinophils following induction by different methods. *Int. Arch. Allergy Appl. Immun.* 1987;**83**:423–427.

9 · Potential involvement of interleukin-5 and platelet-activating factor in eosinophil recruitment in the rat

A. Etienne, D. Hosford, C. Soulard, F. Thonier and P. Braquet*

Introduction

The factors responsible for *in vivo* eosinophil recruitment are poorly defined, although T-lymphocytes appear to be involved in the aetiology of eosinophilia. Recently, studies with the highly selective non-myelotoxic immunosuppressive agent, cyclosporin A (CsA), suggested that this drug, by inhibiting prolactin binding to lymphocytes, is able to decrease the eosinophil recruitment observed in the rat after antigen challenge [1]. Cyclosporin A like the selective platelet-activating factor (PAF) antagonist BN 52021, are drugs that reduce organ transplant rejection [2,3] an activity which may be correlated to their inhibitory effect on eosinophilia. Indeed, eosinophil infiltration into tissues has been observed during corneal [4] or kidney [5] graft rejection in humans and preliminary results in rat allograft skin transplantation demonstrate that BN 52021 also counteracts eosinophil infiltration in this model [6,7]. In addition to its beneficial effects in prevention of graft rejection, BN 52021 also inhibits type I hypersensitivity reactions [reviewed in 8] and decreases the eosinophil recruitment observed in guinea pig [9,10] or rabbit [11] after antigen challenge.

Structurally characterized as 1-O-hexadecyl-2(R)-acetyl-glycero-3-phosphocholine, PAF is an important mediator of anaphylaxis [reviewed in 12,13] and may regulate cell immune responses in various systems [reviewed in 14]. It is highly chemotactic for eosinophils [15], a phenomenon specifically inhibited by BN 52021 [16], and thus could be responsible for the tissue eosinophil infiltration observed in graft rejection or airway hyperreactivity.

Also of interest is the fact that specific receptors for the tetradecapeptide somatostatin have also been identified on lymphocytes and this neuropeptide is known to inhibit T-lymphocyte proliferation [reviewed in 17]. The release of mediators from basophils is also depressed by somatostatin suggesting a role for this peptide in hypersensitivity reactions [reviewed in 17].

In an attempt to clarify the relationships between PAF, eosinophils and the immunological system, we have studied the effects of BN 52021, CsA and somatostatin agonist, BIM 23014, on the granulocyte mobilization induced by antigen challenge

*To whom correspondence should be addressed.

in the peritoneal cavity of the rat. Since the normal rat has a low peripheral eosinophil count relative to allergic humans, rats were made hypereosinophilic by intravenous administration of Sephadex G-200 beads or high-dose cyclophosphamide before the induction of the inflammatory reactions [18].

Materials and methods

Sensitization and challenge

Male Sprague–Dawley rats (220–250 g body weight) were immunized by a subplantar injection in one hind foot of 0.1 ml of a mixture 1:1 volume of ovalbumin in saline solution (2 mg/ml) and complete Freund's adjuvant. The animals were challenged 13 days later by an intraperitoneal injection of 0.5 mg ovalbumin in 0.5 ml saline.

Induction of hypereosinophilia

Animals were either injected intraperitoneally with 150 mg/kg cyclosphosphamide 48 h before immunization [7] or intravenously received 0.5 ml of a 3×10^3 beads/ml Sephadex G-200 suspension in 0.9% NaCl 4 days before challenge [8].

Cell analysis

Animals were killed by terminal ether anaesthesia 4 or 24 h after challenge and the peritoneal cavity of each animal was lavaged with 5 ml of saline containing 6 units/ml heparin. Immediately after, blood samples were removed from the *vena cava.* Total and differential leucocyte counts were determined on blood and peritoneal washings using a Coulter counter and May–Grünwald–Giemsa-stained smears, respectively.

Drugs

The drugs were given daily by oral route (BN 52021 and CsA) or subcutaneously (BIM 23014) from the day of sensitization until day 13, the last administration taking place 1 h before antigen challenge.

BN 52021 (ginkgolide B) was prepared by I.H.B. Research Labs (Le Plessis Robinson, France). BIM 23014 (D-Nal-Cys-Tyr-D-Trp-Lys-Val-Cys-Thr-NH_2) was obtained from Biomeasure Inc (Hopkinton, USA). Cyclosporin A was kindly supplied by Sandoz (Basel, Switzerland).

Results

Effects of BN 52021 and CsA on immune cell mobilization in cyclophosphamide pretreated rats

Peritoneal injection of the antigen in actively sensitized and cyclophosphamide-pretreated rats induced an inflammatory reaction accompanied after 4 h by a marked increase in total leucocyte count of the blood and peritoneal fluid. These variations were still observed, although to a lesser extent, 24 h after challenge (Fig. 9.1). The increase in leucocytes was not significantly modified by chronic treatment with 20 mg/kg/day BN 52021, whereas cyclosporin 25 mg/kg/day strongly reduced leucocyte levels in the blood and in peritoneal fluid. A reduction of about 50% of this cell type was observed (Fig. 9.1).

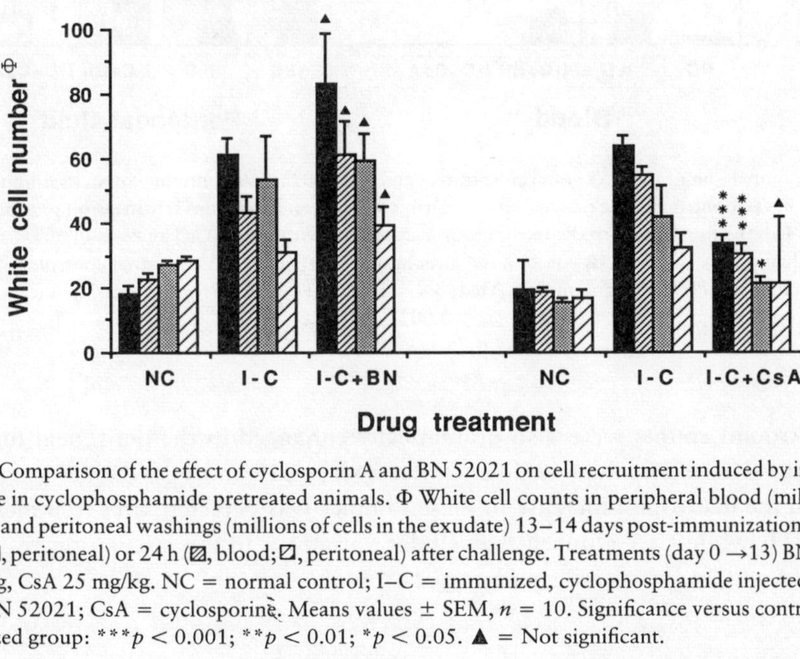

Fig. 9.1. Comparison of the effect of cyclosporin A and BN 52021 on cell recruitment induced by immune challenge in cyclophosphamide pretreated animals. Φ White cell counts in peripheral blood (millions of cells/ml) and peritoneal washings (millions of cells in the exudate) 13–14 days post-immunization, 4 h (■, blood; ▩, peritoneal) or 24 h (▨, blood; ▱, peritoneal) after challenge. Treatments (day 0 →13) BN 52021 20 mg/kg, CsA 25 mg/kg. NC = normal control; I–C = immunized, cyclophosphamide injected (day 2); BN = BN 52021; CsA = cyclosporine. Means values ± SEM, $n = 10$. Significance versus control immunized group: $***p < 0.001$; $**p < 0.01$; $*p < 0.05$. ▲ = Not significant.

Determination of white cell subsets demonstrated that the circulating eosinophil count was markedly enhanced (+400%) 4 h after the immune challenge (Fig. 9.2). This increase was not affected by BN 52021 but totally abolished by cyclosporin, the eosinophil count for this latter drug being below that of the controls. The number of circulating eosinopohils was still higher 24 h after challenge (+550%) (Fig. 9.2). BN 52021 moderately reduced this level (−49%), while the cyclosporin effect was basically the same as that observed after 4 h.

Both BN 52021 and cyclosporin significantly reduced the eosinophil count in the peritoneal exudate both at 4 and 24 h. The value of the BN 52021-treated group was lower than that of the control group and was nil in the peritoneal cavity of CsA-treated animals. The degree of antagonism elicited by the drugs was similar at time 4 h and 24 h (Fig. 9.2).

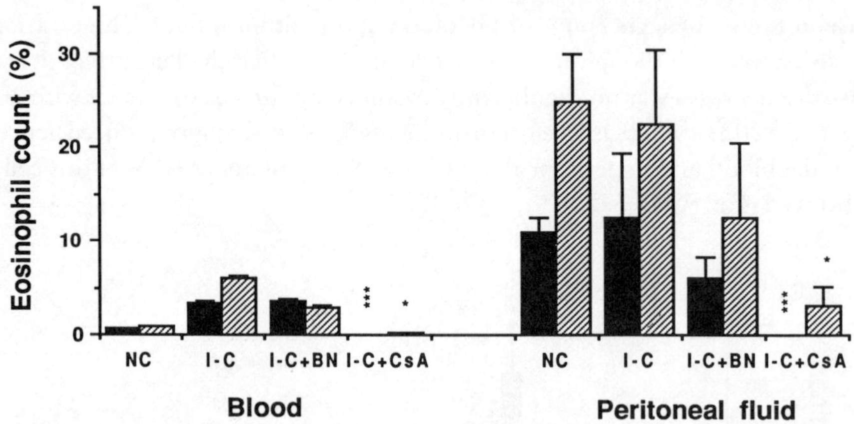

Fig. 9.2. Comparison of the effect of cyclosporin A and BN 52021 on eosinophil count after immune challenge in cyclophosphamide pretreated rats. Drugs were given daily from sensitization to challenge (day 0 → 13); the non-immunized control group was treated with saline. Cell analysis in blood and peritoneal fluid were done 4 h (■) or 24 h (▨) after antigen challenge. NC = normal control; I–C = immunized, cyclophosphamide injected; BN = BN 52021; CsA = cyclosporin. Significance versus control immunized group: $^*p < 0.05$; $^{***}p < 0.001$.

Neutrophil counts were also dramatically enhanced in the peritoneal fluid and blood after 4 h (+290 and +42%) and after 24 h (+210 and +100%). No significant effect on the neutrophil increase in these samples was detected after treatment with BN 52021, while CsA reduced the cellular variations in the circulation by 30 and 55%, at 4 and 24 h respectively (data not shown).

Effect of BIM 23014 on immune mobilization in Sephadex-injected animals

Although the total leucocyte counts were not significantly modified, Sephadex given intravenously 4 days before antigen injection to the rats resulted in a sixfold increase in the number of blood eosinophils 24 h after immune challenge, and a 1.5-fold increase at peritoneal level as compared with the control animals (Fig. 9.3). Neutrophils were increased by 350 and 200% respectively in blood and peritoneal fluid. Chronic treatment with BIM 23014 induced a significant increase of total white cells in the peritoneal washings. This was primarily due to an increase in neutrophil recruitment.

These changes were not observed in the blood. In contrast to the case with neutrophils, the eosinophil mobilization observed in blood as well as in peritoneal fluid 24 h after antigen challenge was significantly decreased by BIM 23014 treatment (−68%, $p < 0.001$ and −86%, $p < 0.5$ respectively). Monocyte depletion in blood or in peritoneal fluid was not significantly modified by this treatment.

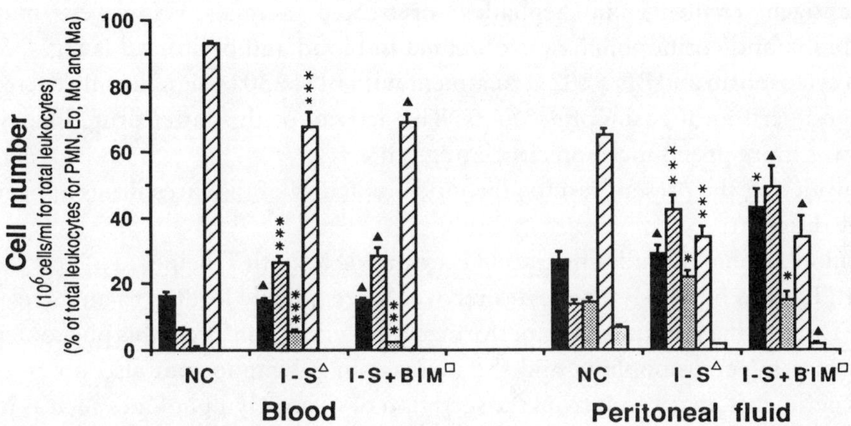

Fig. 9.3. Effect of the somatostatin analogue BIM 23014 on cell mobilization induced by immune challenge in immunized and Sephadex injected animals. Total leucocytes (10^6 cells/ml) and differential cell count (expressed as % of total leucocyte number) for blood and periotoneal fluid were measured 24 h after i.p. antigen injection. (■) Total leucocytes; (▨) neutrophils; (▩) eosinophils; (▨) mononuclear cells; (□) mast-cells. Animals were treated daily with BIM 23014 (10 μg/kg s.c.) or vehicle from day 0 to 13 post-immunization. NC = normal control; I–S = immunized, Sephadex injected; BIM = BIM 23014. Means values ± SEM, $n = 12$. Statistical significance by Student's *t*-test compared with (△) the normal control or (□) to the I–S group. $^{***}p < 0.001$; $^{*}p < 0.05$. ▲ = not significant.

Discussion

Eosinophilia is a well known clinical entity of various aetiologies including allergic states, helminth infestations and in certain cases, graft rejection. Platelet-activating factor and the newly described lymphokine interleukin-5 (IL−5) are potent eosinophil activating factors. In order to clarify the role of these two factors in the mechanism of *in vivo* eosinophilia and eosinophil infiltration, the effects of (i) a PAF antagonist: BN 52021, (ii) cyclosporin, and (iii) a somatostatin analogue: BIM 23014, on cyclophosphamide (or Sephadex)/antigen-induced eosinophilia were investigated. In agreement with the results recently published by Mathie *et al.* [19] chronic administration of cyclosporin from the time of immunization up to the challenge strongly reduced blood eosinophilia, abolished peritoneal eosinophil mobilization and reduced the circulating neutrophil count. BN 52021 also strongly reduced peritoneal eosinophil mobilization but was only slightly effective against the increase in circulating eosinophils and did not modify neutrophil levels.

In the experiment with Sephadex, antigen was injected at day 4, the time of maximum eosinophilia. Sephadex beads alter microvessel endothelium, initiating inflammatory lesions particularly in the lung. Perivascular infiltrations with neutrophils and eosinophils have been observed in this model [20]. In contrast to cyclophosphamide treated animals, no increase in leucocyte count was detected 24 h after antigen challenge in Sephadex pretreated animals. However, marked neutrophilia and eosinophilia were obtained in blood and peritoneal lavages. Similarly to cyclosporin and BN 52021, treatment with BIM 23014 significantly decreased blood and peritoneal eosinophil counts. The activity of this latter drug, like cyclosporin, was more pronounced on circulating cells.

Considering the present results, the mode of action of the three drugs appears to be quite different:

1. Cyclophosphamide administration is cytotoxic to both T-helper (T_H) and T-suppressor (T_s) cells but T_H-lymphocytes recover more quickly leading to an increase in the T_H/T_s ratio; the immunization performed afterwards reinforces this phenomenon. The intense hypereosinophilia and the increase in B-lymphocytes also observed in such experiments, may result from the secretion of various lymphokines such as interleukin-3 (IL-3), granulocyte monocyte-colony stimulating factor (GM-CSF) and IL-5. Indeed, the latter displays the same activity that the lymphokine designated eosinophil differentiation factor (EDF) which also has B-cell growth factor activity (BCGF II) [21,22] and may account for the phenomena observed in this model. Thus, recombinant murine IL-5 (rmIL-5) mimics the activity of the native EDF produced by T_H cells [22] and is also active as a BCGF II [23]. Similarly recombinant human IL-5 (rhIL-5) stimulates eosinophil colony formation but unlike human GM-CSF which also stimulates eosinophil colony formation, no other colony types are produced. In addition, rhIL-5 alters the morphological appearance of eosinophils, a phenomenon related to changes in cytoskeleton occurring after cell activation [24]. It is well established that cyclosporin affects T-cell proliferation and that these cells are involved in the differentiation of haematopoietic cells into eosinophils. The inhibition of IL-5 production by the T_H cells may provide an explanation as to why treatment with this drug affects the eosinophil count of the blood, the decrease in eosinophil mobilization probably reflecting the fact that there are less cells available for recruitment.

2. BIM 23014, as native somatostatin [17], at very low doses ($10^{-14} \rightarrow 10^{-10}$ M) inhibits the proliferation of T-lymphocytes [Pignol and Braquet, unpublished] and therefore may act as cyclosporin, decreasing T_H-cell and the related IL-5 production. In addition, BIM 23014 significantly depresses GH release, a neuropeptide known to exert immuno-enhancing properties [25]. Finally somatostatin has been shown to enhance the formation of human leucocyte migration inhibiting factor [26] an activity which may also account in part for its depressive effect on eosinophils.

3. BN 52021 is a specific PAF antagonist that probably elicits its effect by inhibiting the action of this autacoid on eosinophil chemotaxis, which explains its selective activity at the inflammatory site. In contrast with cyclosporin or BIM 23014, BN 52021 has no direct effect on T_H-cells, only a slight enhancing action of the PAF antagonist on T_s-cells being recorded [27]. Recently, we have elaborated a PAF/cytokine feedback model [28,29] from data showing that PAF and various cytokines can prime and amplify the release of each other and the cytotoxic responses of various inflammatory cells including eosinophils. For example, complex feedback interactions may exist between PAF, TNF and GM-CSF leading to the enhancement of eosinophil cytotoxicity [28,29]. Thus, the effect of the PAF antagonist may also be due to the blockade of PAF/cytokine feedback interactions which would otherwise promote eosinophil recruitment. The inhibitory effect of BN 52021 on eosinophil mobilization may thus explain the beneficial activity of this drug observed in bronchial hyperreactivity and other inflammatory models [reviewed in 8]. The models described in this paper may provide a useful means to investigate drugs able to block eosinophil maturation and/or recruitment, and allow the selection of new treatments for the pathologies in which these cells are operative.

References

1 Hiestand PC, Mekler P, Nordmann R, Grieder A, Permmongkol C. Prolactin as a modulator of lymphocyte responsiveness provides a possible mechanism of action for cyclosporin. *Proc. Natl. Acad. Sci. USA* 1986;83:2599.

2 Kahan BD (Ed.) *Cyclosporin.* Grune & Stratton, Orlando, Florida, 1984.

3 Foegh ML, Khirabadi BS, Rowles JR, Braquet P, Ramwell PW. Prolongation of cardiac allograft survival with BN 52021, a specific antagonist of platelet-activating factor. *Transplantation,* 1986;42:86.

4 Linberg MB, Margo CE, Lyman GH. Eosinophils in corneas removed by penetrating keratoplasty. *Br. J. Ophthalmol.* 1986;70:343.

5 Schlüter E, Lennert K, Bohle A. The immunological significance of cellular infiltrates in chronic rejection of human kidney transplants. *Virchows Arch. A. Pathol. Anat. Histol.* 1975;**368**:191.

6 Bekemeier KO, Lueddeckens, G, Förster, W. Rejection of transplanted mouse skin is delayed by treatment with a prostaglandin analog and a specific PAF antagonist (BN 52021). *Jahrestagung Gesellschaft Pharm. Toxikol. DDR,* January 26–29 1988; (abstract).

7 Rothwell TLW, Papadimitriou JM. The cellular infiltrate in skin allografts in mice. *J. Pathol.* 1972;**107**:235.

8 Braquet P. The Ginkgolides: potent platelet-activating factor antagonists isolated from *Ginkgo biloba* L. Chemistry, pharmacology and clinical applications. *Drugs of the Future* 1987;**12**:643.

9 Coyle AJ, Urwin SC, Page CP, Touvay C, Vilain B, Braquet P. The effect of the selective PAF antagonist BN 52021 on PAF- and antigen-induced bronchial hyper-reactivity and eosinophil accumulation. *Eur. J. Pharmacol.* 1988;**148**:51.

10 Lellouch-Tubiana A, Lefort J, Simon MT, Pfister A, Vargaftig BB. Eosinophil recruitment into guinea-pig lungs after PAF-acether and allergen administration: modulation by prostacyclin, platelet depletion and selective antagonists. *Am. Rev. Resp. Dis.* 1988;**137**:948.

11 Metzger WJ, Sjoerdsma K, Brown L, Coyle T, Page CP, Touvay C. The late phase asthmatic response in the allergic rabbit: a role for platelet-activating factor (PAF) and modification by PAF antagonist,

Ginkgolide BN 52021. In *Ginkgolides, Chemistry, Biology, Pharmacology and Clinical Perspectives,* (Ed. Braquet P), Prous, Barcelona, 1988, p. 313.

12 Braquet P, Touqui L, Shen TY, Vargaftig BB. Perspectives in platelet-activating factor research. *Pharmacol. Rev.* 1987;39:97.

13 Vargaftig BB, Braquet P. PAF-acether today—relevance for acute experimental anaphylaxis. *Br. Med. Bull.* 1987;**43**:312.

14 Braquet P, Rola-Pleszczynski M. Platelet-activating factor and cellular immune responses. *Immunol. Today* 1987;**8**:345.

15 Wardlaw AJ, Moqbel R, Cromwell O, Kay AB. Platelet-activating factor. A potent chemotactic and chemokinetic factor for human eosinophils. *J. Clin. Invest.* 1986;**78**:1701.

16 Tamura N, Agrawal DK, Suliaman FA, Townley RG. Effects of platelet-activating factor on the chemotaxis of normodense eosinophils from normal subjects. *Biochem. Biophys. Res. Com.* 1987;**142**:638.

17 Payan DG, McGillis JP, Goetzl EJ. Neuroimmunology. *Adv. Immunol.* 1986;**39**:299.

18 Thomson AW, Mathie IH, Sewell HF. Cyclophosphamide-induced eosinophilia in the rat: concomitant changes in T-cell subsets, B cells and large granular lymphocytes within lymphoid tissues. *Immunology* 1987;**60**:383.

19 Mathie IH, Sewell HF, Thomson AW. Generation of large granular lymphocytes and lymphocyte subset changes linked with cyclophosphamide-induced eosinophilia in rats—and the effects of ciclosporin. *Scand. J. Immunol.* 1987;**26**:417.

20 Lemanske RF, Kaliner MA. The experimental production of increased eosinophils in rat late-phase reactions. *Immunology* 1982;**45**:561.

21 Azuma T, Tanabe T, Konishi M, Kinashi T, Noma T, Matsuda F, Yaoita Y, Takatsu K, Hammarstrom L, Smith CIE, Severinson E, Honjo T. Cloning of cDNA for human T-cell replacing factor (interleukin-5) and comparison with the murine homologue. *Nucleic Acids Res.* 1986;**14**:9149.

22 Yamaguchi Y, Suda T, Suda J, Eguchi M, Miura Y, Harada N, Tominage A, Takatsu K. Purified interleukin-5 supports the terminal differentiation and proliferation of murine eosinophilic precursors. *J. Exp. Med.* 1988;**167**:43.

23 Alderson MR, Pike BL, Harada N, Tominage A, Takatsu K, Nossal GJV. Recombinant T cell replacing factor (interleukin-5) acts with antigen to promote the growth and differentiation of single hapten-specific B lymphocytes. *J. Immunol.* 1987;**8**:2656.

24 Campbell HD, Tucker WQJ, Hort Y, Martinson ME, Mayo G, Clutterbuck EJ, Sanderson CJ, Young IG. Molecular cloning and expression of the gene encoding human eosinophil differentiation factor (interleukin-5). *Proc. Natl. Acad. Sci. USA* 1987;**84**:6629.

25 Gupta S, Fikrig SM, Noval MS. Immunological studies in patients with isolated growth hormone deficiency. *Clin. Exp. Immunol.* 1983;**54**:87.

26 Pawlikowski M, Zelazowski P, Stepien H, Schally AV. Somatostatin and its analog enhance the formation of human leukocyte migration inhibiting factor: further evidence of immunomodulatory action of somatostatin. *Peptides* 1987;**8**:951.

27 Rola-Pleszczynski M, Pouliot C, Turcotte S, Pignol B, Braquet P, Bouvrette L. PAF induces human helper and suppressor cells. *J. Immunol.* 1988;**104**:3547.

28 Braquet P, Braquet M, Koltai M, Bourgain R, Bussolino F, Hosford D. Viewpoint: is there a case for PAF antagonists in the treatment of ischemic states? *TIPS* 1989;**10**:23–30.

29 Braquet P, Paubert-Braquet M, Bourgain RH, Bussolino F, Hosford D. PAF/cytokine auto-generated feedback networks in microvascular immune injury: consequences in shock, ischemia and graft rejection. *J. Lipid Mediators* 1989;**1**:75–112.

10 · The role of neutrophils and eosinophils in a model of asthma in the guinea pig

S.T. Holgate,* Penny A. Hutson, Janis K. Shute, S. Janet Rimmer, Catherine L. Akerman and M.K. Church

Introduction

Studies on the mechanisms of the late asthmatic response (LAR) and acquired bronchial hyperresponsiveness (BHR) have become increasingly important areas of study in understanding the pathophysiological mechanisms of bronchial asthma. Bronchial provocation of extrinsic asthmatic subjects induces an early asthmatic response (EAR), which peaks at 15–30 min and is mediated by the actions of inflammatory mast cell-derived mediators [1]. In a large proportion of subjects this is followed by a LAR which begins 4–12 h after challenge and lasts for several hours [2]. The onset of the LAR is accompanied by the acquisition of increased responsiveness of the airways to non-specific stimulation [3]. Clear differences between the mechanisms of the EAR and the LAR in man have been demonstrated by their susceptibility to blockade by anti-asthmatic drugs; anti-allergic drugs such as sodium cromoglycate (SCG) and nedocromil sodium blocking both the EAR and the LAR [2,4,5] while beta-adrenoceptor stimulants inhibit only the EAR [5,6] and corticosteroids only the LAR [5,7].

The inflammatory basis of the LAR is illustrated by the recovery of increased numbers of neutrophils and eosinophils from the airways by bronchoalveolar lavage (BAL) [8,9]. Although both granulocytes contain inflammatory mediators within their secretory granules, evidence is accumulating for a role of the eosinophil rather than the neutrophil in allergic responses [10]. Unlike the neutrophil, the eosinophil possesses cell surface receptors for IgE (FcεRII) which enable it to interact with allergen in IgE-dependent reactions [11,12]. When activated eosinophils have the potential to generate the potent bronchoconstrictor agent, leukotriene (LT) C_4 [13], platelet-activating factor (PAF) [14] and reactive species of oxygen [15]. In addition, they may release their preformed granule-associated proteins including major basic protein (MBP) [16] and eosinophil cationic protein (ECP) [8], both of which have been associated with cellular damage in the lung [5,17].

The presence in the circulation of hypodense eosinophils indicative of cellular immaturity or partial degranulation, in late responses [18], also the demonstration that eosinophils are recovered from the lung by BAL during the late response [8] and

*To whom correspondence should be addressed.

the demonstration of eosinophil derived proteins in the sputum of asthmatic subjects [19], all incriminate the eosinophil in the pathogenesis of the later phases of the asthmatic response.

In this review we describe experiments in the guinea pig *in vivo* designed to explore the mechanism of the late response and *in vitro* studies on the activation of guinea pig eosinophils.

Models of the late response in the guinea pig

Because of the ethical limitations involved in the study of LAR and the acquisition of BHR in man, a number of models have been developed in experimental animals including sheep [20], rabbits [21], rats [22] and squirrel monkeys [23].

The traditional immunological model of antigen-induced airway obstruction has been the guinea pig. The actively immunized guinea pig challenged systemically with antigen develops anaphylaxis, which is often fatal. As long ago as 1910, Auer and Lewis [24] attributed this fatal anaphylaxis to severe bronchoconstriction. Similarities exist between guinea pigs and humans in the response to a variety of contractile and relaxant substances, in the putative involvement of chemical mediators in antigen-induced responses [25] and in the histopathological changes that occur in the lungs following antigen challenge [26]. The main homocytotropic antibody in the guinea pig, however, is IgG [27]. This fact, and the conflicting results that have been obtained with the effects of sodium cromoglycate (SCG) on antigen-induced airways obstruction have made the guinea pig a less widely used animal in the testing of anti-allergic drugs [28]. The finding, however, that suitably sensitized guinea pigs are capable of producing IgE-like antibodies [29,30] has created further interest in this species as a model of human asthma.

Until recently there have been no descriptions of late-phase responses within the lungs in the guinea pig. The realization of the potential importance of the LAR to the investigation of clinical asthma has led investigators to attempt to produce these responses in this species. Wieslander *et al.* [31] described a model in which guinea pigs were systemically sensitized with ovalbumin to preferentially produce IgE rather than IgG antibodies. Provocation of animals by intratracheal instillation of soluble ovalbumin produced severe early responses but did not provoke late-phase responses. However, instillation into the trachea of ovalbumin covalently linked to sepharose beads resulted in a second phase of increased airways resistance, which reached a maximum 20 h after challenge. Bronchoalveolar lavage (BAL) performed in guinea pigs exhibiting a LAR revealed a significantly raised number of neutrophils and eosinophils, and histological examination of the lungs revealed focal inflammation around the sepharose beads deposited in the bronchioles.

Iijima *et al.* [32] described a model of the LAR in which guinea pigs were systemically sensitized with a mixture of *Ascaris suum* extract and aluminium hydroxide.

Following inhalation challenge with an aerosol of the parasite extract, approximately half of the guinea pigs studied developed a late response 6–8 h after challenge. Bronchoalveolar lavage performed during the LAR showed a marked neutrophilia that did not differ significantly from that seen in animals which only showed an EAR. Histological sections, however, showed a more prominent eosinophil infiltration into the airway walls of animals exhibiting a LAR. In addition, contraction of airway smooth-muscle, submucosal oedema and secretion of mucus into the airway lumen were observed, features which were not seen in the model described by Wieslander *et al.* [31].

There are several disadvantages associated with the animal models described above. The main disadvantage of the model described by Iijima *et al.* [32] is the inconsistency of the response. In the model described by Wieslander *et al.* [31], instillation of sepharose beads alone induces an accumulation of neutrophils in the airways. Further, the use of anaesthetic in the measurement of pulmonary function may suppress important neuronal reflexes and precludes the ability to perform repeated measurements over long periods of time. Perhaps most importantly in both these models, sensitization is achieved by parenteral (intraperitoneal and/or subcutaneous) injection of allergen to induce systemic sensitization. In humans, the natural route of sensitization is by inhalation of airborne allergens.

In an effort to overcome some of the practical problems associated with other methods, we have developed a model of early and late-phase airways changes in the guinea pig in which animals are sensitized and challenged by inhalation of allergen and lung function is measured in conscious animals by whole body plethysmography [33]. Male Dunkin Hartley guinea pigs are actively sensitized by inhalation of 10 mg/ml ovalbumin aerosol for 3 min on days 0 and 7. To assess early and late-phase responses to challenge, guinea pigs inhale 20 mg/ml ovalbumin on day 14 for 5 min under the protection of a histamine H_1-antagonist, mepyramine maleate (10 mg/kg) injected intraperitoneally 30 min before challenge. The use of a histamine H_1-antagonist protects the animals from the potentially lethal effects of large amounts of histamine released during the early response [34] and allows the administration of a sufficiently high dose of antigen to provoke reproducible late responses. Specific airways conductance (sGaw) (airways conductance at unit thoracic gas volume) is measured in conscious animals by whole body plethysmography both before challenge and at repeated intervals up to 72 h after challenge [33]. In experiments to determine bronchial hyperresponsiveness, the effect of histamine and methacholine on bronchial function may also be assessed by whole body plethysmography at day 14. Infiltration of the airways with inflammatory cells is quantified by counting the leucocytes recovered by BAL at various intervals following challenge. In addition, at selected time points, samples of airways tissue are prepared for examination by light and electron microscopy [33].

Sensitization and antigen provocation of guinea pigs

Sensitization of guinea pigs led to a 4.1- and 1.6-fold decrease in the concentrations of histamine and methacholine respectively required to cause a 20% fall in sGaw from baseline. This was accompanied by a 3.3-fold increase in the number of eosinophils recovered by BAL suggesting a possible relationship between this cell and acquired hyperresponsiveness [35].

Antigen provocation of sensitized guinea pigs induced three phases of increased airways resistance [33]; an early response occurring within 5 min and reaching a maximum at 2 h, a second or late response peaking at 17 h and a further late response which is evident at 72 h (Fig. 10.1). The early response was dominated by an increase in thoracic gas volume, indicative of air trapping within the airways compared with the two late responses which were dominated by increases in airways resistance. Inhalation of saline by sensitized guinea pigs produced no significant changes in sGaw from baseline (Fig. 10.1).

Examination of cells recovered from BAL revealed an influx of both neutrophils and eosinophils into the airways [36]. Neutrophil numbers were maximal at 17 h and returned to near baseline levels by 72 h. Eosinophil accumulation, however, was more gradual, beginning at 6 h after challenge and still increasing at 72 h when these cells constituted 48.9±6.9% of the total leucocyte population (Fig. 10.2). Further experiments have shown that eosinophil numbers were still significantly greater in ovalbumin-challenged animals when compared with saline-challenged animals, at 7 days, although absolute numbers were lower than at 72 h.

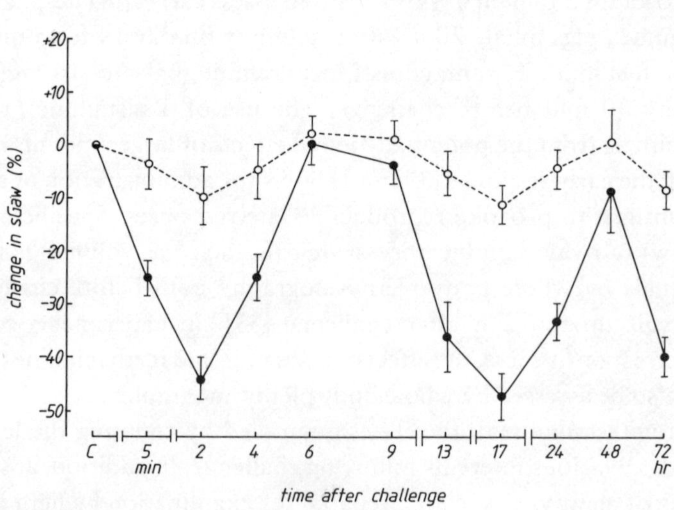

Fig. 10.1. The effect of saline control (○——○) and ovalbumin (2%) (●- - -●) inhalation on specific airways conductance (sGaw) in sensitized guinea pigs.

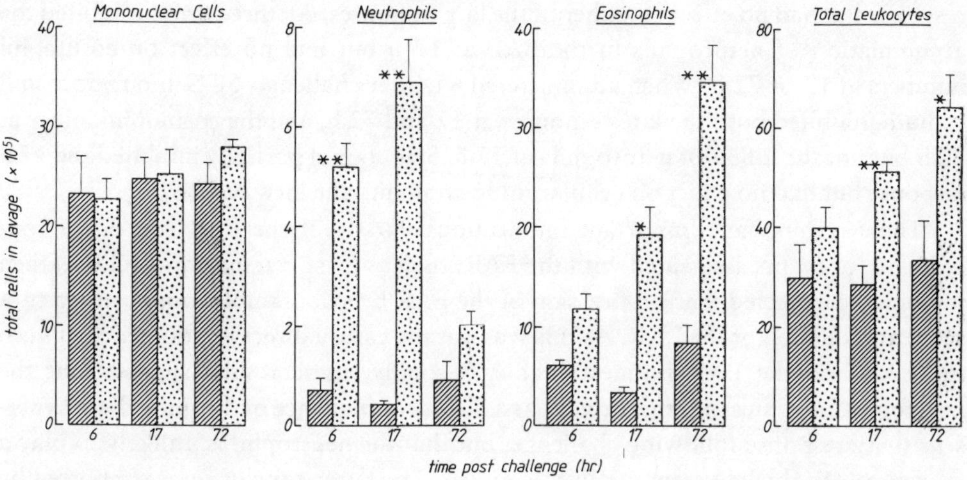

Fig. 10.2. Differential leucocyte counts in BAL from saline control (hatched bars) and ovalbumin (2%) (stippled bars) challenged guinea pigs. * and ** indicate statistical significance ($p < 0.05$ and $p < 0.01$ respectively).

Histopathological examination of tracheal and lung sections by light microscopy revealed an infiltration of polymorphonuclear leucocytes within the airways of animals challenged with ovalbumin which was not seen in controls. At 17 and 72 h this leucocyte infiltration was dominated by eosinophils which were present beneath and between the epithelial cells and was seen to be tracking through channels in the smooth-muscle. The cellular infiltration was confined to the airways and was not present in the alveoli. Electron microscopical examination of tracheal epithelium at 17 h after challenge confirmed the presence of eosinophils beneath and in between the epithelial cells and further showed some loss of the electron dense crystalloid core of the granules, suggesting that they had been activated for secretion. In addition, a dramatic degranulation of goblet cells was observed indicating that mucus secretion had occurred. Electron microscopical examination of eosinophils from BAL fluid at 17 h also revealed a loss of core material from the granules.

Pharmacological manipulation of allergen-induced early and late responses and airway leucocyte infiltration

For an animal model of asthma to be relevant to the clinical situation, a similar profile of drug activity should be demonstrable. In our guinea pig model we have observed this to be the case. Inhalation of SCG (10 mg/ml) or nedocromil sodium (10 mg/ml) by sensitized guinea pigs 15 min before challenge, inhibited both the early response and the late response at 17 h, but not the 72-h response. In contrast, inhalation of the β_2-adrenoceptor agonist, salbutamol (0.1 mg/ml) before challenge inhibits the early response but had no effect on either of the late responses. All three drugs inhibited the accumulation of neturophils in the BAL at 17 h but had no effect on eosinophil numbers at 17 or 72 h. When administered 6 h after challenge, SCG and nedocromil sodium inhibited both the late responses at 17 and 72 h, and the eosinophil influx at 72 h but not the influx of neturophils at 17 h. Salbutamol partially inhibited the 17 h response but had no effect on cellular infiltration into the airways [36,37].

These results have important implications. Firstly, if the LAR is a direct consequence of events associated with the EAR, such as mast-cell mediator release, then it would be expected that suppression of the EAR by salbutamol would cause a subsequent reduction of the LAR. As this was not the case, a direct relationship between the EAR and the LAR is questionable. Secondly, these results suggest that the neutrophil infiltrates into the airways as a direct consequence of the immediate hypersensitivity response following challenge, but that the neutrophil is unlikely to play a crucial role in the late response in this model. The latter conclusion is supported by experiments in which pretreatment of guinea pigs with an anti-neutrophil serum did not affect the late response at 17 h despite abolishing the influx of neutrophils into the lung at this time [38].

The role of the eosinophil in the late response in this guinea pig model is not yet clear. There is no clear relationship between the numbers of eosinophils recovered in BAL and the presence of a LAR, eosinophil numbers rising slowly between 6 and 72 h whereas the late airways response occurs at 17 h after challenge [33]. Furthermore, the late response at 17 h can be inhibited by inhalation of SCG or nedocromil sodium either before or after challenge without a parallel effect on eosinophil numbers at this time. In contrast, there appears to be a temporal relationship between the late airways response at 72 h and accumulation of eosinophils at this time since both SCG and nedocromil inhibited this response with a parallel reduction in eosinophil numbers. However, conclusions using BAL cytology are limited as they do not take into consideration cell activation and do not allow for the transit time between cell diapedesis from the blood vessels and their appearance in BAL. As described above, data from electron microscopical examination of the lung would argue in favour of the participation of the eosinophil in the LAR.

The inflammatory mediator, PAF, which is not only released from human eosinophils [14] but is also a potent chemotactic agent for these cells [39], has recently been demonstrated to have a number of properties appropriate to a mediator of asthma [40]. Administration of PAF to a number of experimental animals including the guinea pig elicits a selective eosinophilia in the lungs. Furthermore, recent observations have shown that allergen-induced eosinophil accumulation in the airways of experimental animals may be abrogated by PAF antagonists [41]. In addition, the PAF antagonists BN 52063 or WEB 2086 administered prior to challenge have been shown to attenuate the late-phase pulmonary response [42,43]. In our guinea pig model oral administration of WEB 2086 (0.5 mg/kg) prior to allergen challenge shortened the duration of the EAR and the late response peaking at 17 h, and reduced the eosinophil influx at this time [44]. WEB 2086 administered between the early and late-phase responses at 6 h after challenge completely inhibited both late responses at 17 and 72 h and reduced the eosinophil accumulation at 72 h. Although WEB 2086 has a duration of action of only 3–4 h in the guinea pig, these results provide some evidence that PAF is a chemotactic mediator for the recruitment of eosinophils and furthermore suggest that PAF may be of major importance in initiating late responses in this model.

Evidence for activation of eosinophils in the guinea pig

There is growing interest in the findings that in many human conditions associated with eosinophilia, including late-phase asthma [18] and allergic rhinitis [45] there is a population of hypodense or light density eosinophils. These eosinophils show morphological signs of degranulation and a low content of granular MBP [46] and ECP [47] consistent with the hypothesis that these cells have been activated for secretion. It has also been shown that IgE-dependent release of eosinophil peroxidase (EPO) was restricted to hypodense eosinophils [48]. Hence the degree of eosinophil activation and degranulation is likely to be more important in the development of bronchial hyperreactivity than just the presence *per se* of eosinophils in the airways.

In the guinea pig model described above, studies of the density profile of eosinophils in BAL fluid showed a heterogeneous population of cells. In contrast eosinophils derived by peritoneal lavage of animals sensitized intraperitoneally with horse serum showed a homogeneous population of eosinophils (Fig. 10.3) with a

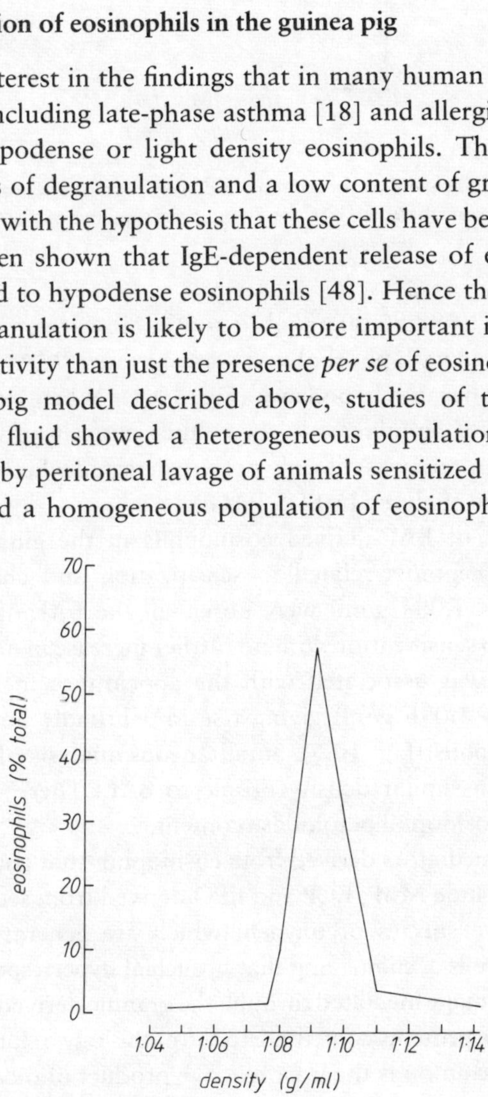

Fig. 10.3. A representative density profile of guinea pig peritoneal eosinophils isolated by continuous density gradient centrifugation on Percoll.

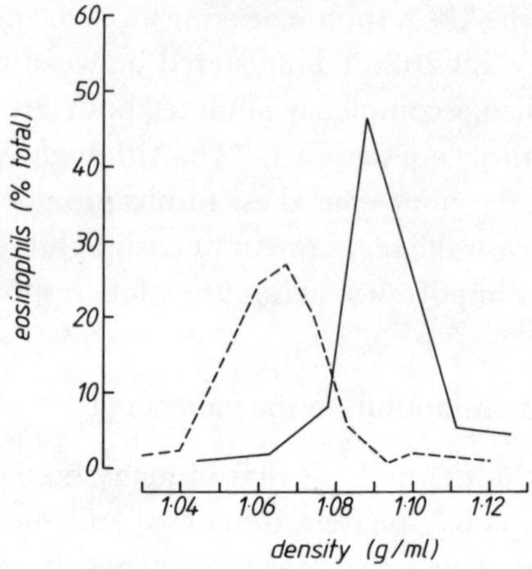

Fig. 10.4. The effect of PMA (1 μg/ml) on the continuous density profile of peritoneal eosinophils from one guinea pig. Eosinophils were incubated at 37°C for 3 min in the presence of PMA (- - - - -) or 0.2% DMSO (————) as control.

mean peak density of 1.088±0.004 g/ml (n = 10). However, when these peritoneal eosinophils were treated with phorbol myristate acetate (PMA) at a final concentration of 1 μg/ml they became hypodense (Fig. 10.4). When examined by electron microscopy they showed an increase in the volume per cent of vacuoles in the cytoplasma. Major basic protein was the only protein detected when supernatants of cells treated with PMA were analysed by SDS-PAGE.

The heterogeneity of BAL-derived eosinophils in the guinea pig model, was studied at specific timepoints related to sensitization and challenge. Hypodense eosinophils (density < 1.084 g/ml) were absent in the BAL of naïve animals and appeared in relation to sensitization with no further increase in numbers after antigen challenge. Challenge was associated with the appearance in BAL of hyperdense eosinophils (density > 1.096 g/ml) giving rise to a broadly heterogeneous density distribution of eosinophils (Fig. 10.5). Simultaneous analysis of tracheal and bronchial digests showed a similar density profile to BAL. There was no relationship between density and eosinophil peroxidase content.

Proinflammatory mediators derived from eosinophils that could contribute to the late-phase reaction include MBP, ECP and EPO derived from secretory granules and LTC_4, PAF and active species of oxygen, which are generated and released by activated cells. Evidence is accumulating that bronchial hyperresponsiveness is secondary to epithelial cell damage mediated through the granule derived proteins MBP, ECP and EPO and that these proteins contribute to the pathology of fatal bronchial asthma [49]. While superoxide anion is the least reactive product of oxygen metabolism, its dismutation to hydrogen peroxide generates the substrate for EPO and is, therefore, a source of the highly reactive hypohalous acids. Concomitant release of EPO

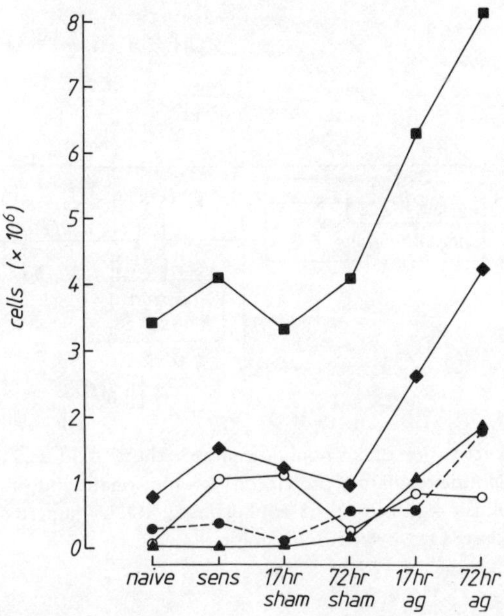

Fig. 10.5. Absolute numbers of cells recovered from BAL fluid after sensitization and challenge of guinea pig lungs with ovalbumin (ag) or saline (sham). Eosinophils were isolated on continuous density gradients of Percoll. Total cells in BAL (■——■); eosinophils total (♦——♦); hyperdense, $p > 1.096$ g/ml, eosinophils (▲——▲); normodense, $p = 1.080–1.096$ g/ml, eosinophils (●---●); hypodense, $p < 1.080$ g/ml, eosinophils (○——○). Each point represents the mean of 4–11 determinations.

in response to agonists of superoxide production therefore would establish conditions for formation of potentially harmful, tissue damaging products of oxygen metabolism.

The number of eosinophils derived by peritoneal lavage is at least 10-fold greater than that obtained by BAL of a single animal. Therefore our *in vitro* studies have concentrated on the mechanism of activation of guinea pig peritoneal eosinophils using the release of EPO and the generation of reactive species of oxygen as indicators of activation. Peritoneal eosinophilia was induced by biweekly intraperitoneal injections of 0.5 ml of horse serum for 2 weeks and maintained by weekly injections of horse serum. Cells were recovered by peritoneal lavage under methoxyfluorane anaesthesia and the animals allowed to recover thus permitting repeated lavage. Lavage fluid contained approximately 30% eosinophils which were purified to > 95% homogeneity on discontinuous gradients of Percoll. The hypothesis we tested was that following receptor occupancy by extracellular stimuli polyphosphoinositide metabolism via a guanine nucleotide regulating protein (Gp) is initiated. This mechanism of stimulus–response coupling is found in many cell types, including neutrophils [50]. Phospholipase-C mediated hydrolysis of the polyphosphoinositides of cell plasma membranes generates diacylglycerol (DAG), an activator of protein

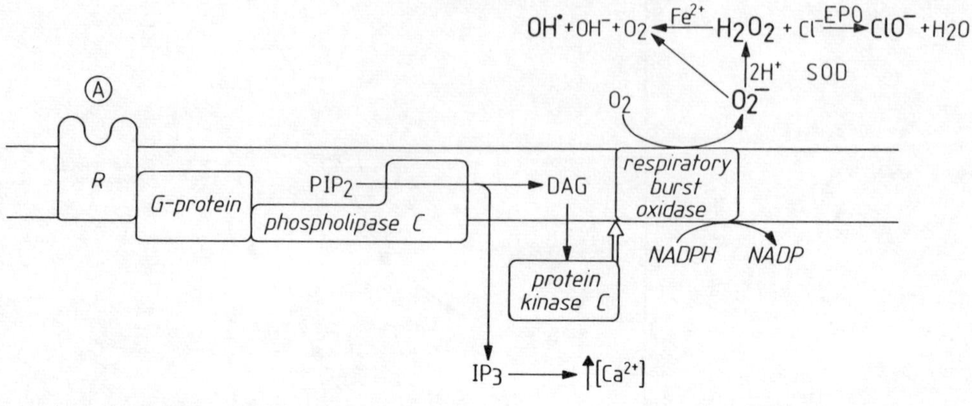

Fig. 10.6. A model for the activation of eosinophil respiratory burst oxidase. A = agonist; R = receptor; G-protein = guanine nucleotide regulatory protein; PIP_2 = phosphatidylinositol 4,5-biphosphate; DAG = 1,2-diacylglycerol; IP_3 = inositol 1,4,5-triphosphate; SOD = superoxide dismutase; EPO = eosinophil peroxidase; O_{-2} = superoxide anion.

kinase C, at a site where it could be responsible for activation of the respiratory burst oxidase. However, a variety of agonists stimulate the oxidase and there may be several activation pathways some of which are dependent on phospholipase A_2 (PLA_2) mediated lipid hydrolysis and independent of protein kinase C [51]. Phospholipase A_2-mediated reactions are activated via G-proteins [52] and generate arachidonic acid which may directly or indirectly stimulate the oxidase. We initially investigated our hypothesis in an indirect manner. Peritoneal eosinophils were exposed to a variety of potential agonists of superoxide production acting sequentially in the proposed pathway (Fig. 10.6). Opsonized zymosan (OPZ) was the receptor-directed agonist used in the study, sodium fluoride was employed as a universal G-protein activator, digitonin as a non-receptor directed activator of phospholipase-C mediated phosphoinositide hydrolysis, the calcium ionophore A23187 as an activator of PLA_2 and phorbol ester as an activator of protein kinase C. Superoxide production in response to the agonists was inhibited by trifluoperazine (TFP), an inhibitor of protein kinase C. The phospholipase inhibitor mepacrine, however, abolished the response to all the agonists except phorbol ester, confirming that the site of action of the phorbol ester was distal to phospholipid hydrolysis. These results indicated that eosinophil activation and superoxide production occurred through mechanisms of phospholipid hydrolysis and protein phosphorylation.

When EPO or arylsulphatase (AS) release were used as a marker of cell activation the cells were completely refractory not only to opsonized zymosan, A23187, sodium fluoride, digitonin and PMA but also to PAF, which we also have shown to stimulate superoxide production. This could indicate that exocytosis of EPO and generation of superoxide are unlikely to occur simultaneously *in vivo* and may represent a control mechanism on the potentially damaging parallel release of EPO and superoxide. Since the granule core protein MBP was released by PMA, which failed to release the matrix protein EPO and the small granule protein AS a specific degranulation mechanism for MBP is indicated.

Our *in vivo* and *in vitro* guinea pig studies of the functions of granulocytes in late-phase allergic responses and bronchial hyperresponsiveness have indicated the potential importance of the eosinophil in this experimental model. Although fundamental differences may exist between the cellular changes in animal models such as those we describe in the guinea pig and human asthma, they have helped considerably in defining the complex cellular interactions involved in allergic tissue responses and have provided clues about the mechanisms of anti-asthma drugs.

References

1 Holgate ST, Benyon RC, Howarth PH, Agius R, Hardy C, Robinson C, Durham SR, Kay AB, Church MK. Relationship between mediator release from human lung mast cells *in vitro* and *in vivo*. *Int. Arch. Allergy Appl. Immunol.* 1985;77:47–56.

2 Pepys J, Hutchcroft BJ. Bronchial provocation tests in etiologic diagnosis and analysis of asthma. *Am. Rev. Respir. Dis.* 1975;**112**:829–859.

3 Cartier A, Thomson NC, Frith PA, Roberts R, Hargreave FE. Allergen-induced increase in bronchial responsiveness to histamine: relationship to the late asthmatic response and change in airway calibre. *J. Allergy Clin. Immunol.* 1982;**70**:170–177.

4 Holgate ST. Clinical evaluation of nedocromil sodium in the treatment of asthma. *Eur. J. Respir. Dis.* 1986;**69** (Suppl. 147):149–159.

5 Cockcroft DW, Murdock KY. Comparative effects of inhaled salbutamol, sodium cromoglycate, and beclomethasone dipropionate on allergen-induced early asthmatic responses, late asthmatic responses, increased bronchial responsiveness to histamine. *J. Allergy Clin. Immunol.* 1987;**79**:734–740.

6 Hegardt B, Pauwels R, van der Straeten M. Inhibitory effect of KWD 2131, terbutaline, and DSCG on the immediate and late allergen-induced bronchoconstriction. *Allergy* 1981;**36**:115–122.

7 Booij Noord H, Orie NGM, de Vries K. Immediate and late bronchial obstructive reactions to inhalation of house dust and protective effects of disodium cromoglycate and prednisolone. *J. Allergy Clin. Immunol.* 1971;**48**:344–354.

8 de Monchy JGR, Kauffman HF, Venge P, Koeter GH, Jansen HM, Sluiter HJ, de Vries K. Broncho alveolar eosinophilia during allergen-induced late asthmatic reactions. *Am. Rev. Respir. Dis.* 1985;**131**:373–376.

9 Metzger WJ, Richerson HB, Worden K, Monick M, Hunninghake GW. Bronchoalveolar lavage of allergic asthmatic patients following allergen provocation. *Chest* 1986;**89**:477–483.

10 Durham SR, Kay AB. Eosinophils, bronchial hyperreactivity and late-phase asthmatic reactions. *Clin. Allergy* 1985;**15**:411–418.

11 Capron M, Jouault T, Prin L, Joseph M, Ameisen JC, Butterworth AE, Papin JP, Kusnierz JP, Capron A. Functional study of a monoclonal antibody to IgE Fc receptor (FcεR2) of eosinophils, platelets and macrophages. *J. Exp. Med.* 1986;**164**:72–89.

12 Walsh GM, Kay AB. Binding of immunoglobulin classes and subclasses to human eosinophils and neutrophils. *Clin. Exp. Immunol.* 1986;**63**:466–472.

13 Jorg A, Henderson WR, Murphy RC, Klebanoff J. Leukotriene generation by eosinophils. *J. Exp. Med.* 1982;**155**:390–402.

14 Lee TC, Lenihan DJ, Malone B, Ruddy LL, Wasserman SI. Increased synthesis of platelet activating factor in activated human eosinophils. *J. Biol. Chem.* 1984;**259**:5526–5530.

15 Venge P. Eosinophil and neutrophil granulocytes in asthma. In *Glucocorticosteriods, Inflammation and Bronchial Hyperreactivity* (Eds Hogg JC, Ellul-Micallef R, Brattsand R), Excerpta Medica, Amsterdam, 1984; pp. 21–37.
16 Lewis DM, Lewis JC, Loegering DA, Gleich GJ. Localization of the guinea-pig eosinophil major basic protein to the core of the granule. *J. Cell Biol.* 1978;77:702–713.
17 Frigas E, Gleich GJ. The eosinophil and the pathophysiology of asthma. *J. Allergy Clin. Immunol.* 1986;77:527–537.
18 Frick WE, Sedgwick JB, Busse WW. The appearance of hypodense eosinophils (HE) in late phase asthma. *J. Allergy Clin. Immunol.* 1988;**81**:208.
19 Filley WV, Holley KE, Kephart GM, Gleich GJ. Identification by immunofluorescence of eosinophil granule major basic protein in lung tissue of patients with bronchial asthma. *Lancet* 1982;**ii**:11–16.
20 Abraham WM, Delehunt JC, Yerger L, Marchette B. Characterization of a late phase pulmonary response following antigen challenge in allergic sheep. *Am. Rev. Respir. Dis.* 1983;**128**:839–844.
21 Shampain MP, Behrens BL, Larsen GL, Henson PM. An animal model of late pulmonary responses to Alternaria challenge. *Am. Rev. Respir. Dis.* 1983;**126**:493–498.
22 Eidelman DH, Bellofiore S, Martin JG. Late airway responses to antigen challenge in sensitised inbred rats. *Am. Rev. Respir. Dis.* 1988;**137**:1033–1037.
23 Hamel R, McFarlane CS, Ford-Hutchinson AW. Late pulmonary responses induced by *Ascaris* allergen in conscious squirrel monkeys. *J. Appl. Physiol.* 1986;**61**:2081–2087.
24 Aver J, Lewis PA. The physiology of the immediate reaction of anaphylaxis in the guinea pig. *J. Exp. Med.* 1910;**12**:151–175.
25 Collier HOJ, James GWL. Humoral factors affecting pulmonary inflation during acute anaphylaxis in the guinea pig *in vivo*. *Br. J. Pharmacol. Chemother.* 1967;**30**:283–301.
26 Kallos P, Kallos L. Experimental asthma in guinea-pigs revisited. *Int. Arch. Allergy Appl. Immunol.* 1984;**73**:77–85.
27 Perini A, Mota I. Heterogenicity of guinea-pig homocytotropic antibodies. *Immunology* 1972;**22**:915–923.
28 Church MK. Cromoglycate-like anti-allergic drugs. *Drugs of Today* 1978;**14**:281–341.
29 Ovary Z, Kaplan B, Kojima S. Characteristics of guinea pig IgE. *Int. Arch. Allergy Appl. Immunol.* 1976;**51**:416–428.
30 Andersson P. Antigen-induced bronchial anaphylaxis in actively sensitized guinea-pigs. Pattern of response in relation to immunization regimen. *Allergy* 1980;**35**:65–71.
31 Wieslander E, Andersson P, Linden M, Axelsson B, Kallstrom L, Brattsand R, Paulsson I. Importance of particulate antigen for the induction of dual bronchial reaction in guinea-pigs. *Agents Actions* 1985;**16**:37–38.
32 Iijima H, Ishii M, Yamauchi K, Chao CL, Kimura K, Shimura S, Shindoh Y, Inoue H, Mue S, Takishima T. Bronchoalveolar lavage and histologic characterization of late asthmatic response in guinea pigs. *Am. Rev. Respir. Dis.* 1987;**136**:922–929.
33 Hutson PA, Church MK, Clay TP, Miller P, Holgate ST. Early and late phase bronchoconstriction following allergen challenge of non-anaesthetized guinea pigs: I. The association of disordered airway physiology to leucocyte infiltration. *Am. Rev. Respir. Dis.* 1988;**137**:548–557.
34 Adams GK, Lichtenstein LM. *In vitro* studies of antigen-induced bronchospasm: effect of antihistamine and SRS-A antagonist on response of sensitized guinea pig and human airways to antigen. *J. Immunol.* 1979;**122**:555–562.
35 Featherstone RL, Hutson PA, Holgate ST, Church MK. Active sensitization of guinea-pig airways *in vivo* enhances *in vivo* and *in vitro* responsiveness. *Eur. J. Respir. Dis.* 1988;**1**:839–845.
36 Hutson PA, Holgate ST, Church MK. The effect of cromolyn sodium and albuterol on early and late phase bronchoconstriction and airway leukocyte infiltration following allergen challenge of non-anaesthetized guinea-pigs. *Am. Rev. Respir. Dis.* 1988a;**138**:1157–1163.
37 Hutson PA, Holgate ST, Church MK. Inhibition by nedocromil sodium of early and late bronchoconstriction and airways cellular infiltration provoked by ovalbumin in conscious sensitized guinea-pigs. *Br. J. Pharmacol.* 1988b;**94**:6.

38 Hutson PA, Sanjar S, Kings M, Holgate ST, Church MK. Evidence that neutrophils do not participate in the late phase airways response provoked by ovalbumin inhalation in conscious sensitized guinea-pigs. *Am. Rev. Respir. Dis.* 1989 (in press).
39 Wardlaw A, Moqbel R, Cromwell O, Kay AB. Platelet-activating factor: A potent chemotactic and chemokinetic factor for eosinophils. *J. Clin. Invest.* 1986;**78**:1701–1706.
40 Braquet P, Touqui L, Shen TY, Vargaftig BB. Perspectives in platelet-activating factor research. *Pharmacol. Rev.* 1987;**39**:97–145.
41 Lellouch-Tubiana A, Lefort J, Simon M–T, Pfister A, Vargaftig BB. Eosinophil recruitment into guinea-pig lungs after PAF-acether and allergen administration. *Am. Rev. Respir. Dis.* 1988;**137**:948–954.
42 Coyle A, Sjoerdsma K, Page CP, Brown L, Metzger WJ. Modification of the late asthmatic response and bronchial hyperreactivity by BN 52021, a platelet activating factor antagonist. *Clin. Res.* 1987;**35**:A254.
43 Stevenson JS, Tallent M, Blinder L, Abraham WM. Modification of antigen-induced late responses with an antagonist of platelet activating factor (WEB 2086) (abstract). *Fed. Proc.* 1987;**46**:1416.
44 Hutson PA, Holgate ST, Church MK. Effect of WEB-2086 on early and late airways responses to ovalbumin challenge in conscious guinea-pigs (abstract). *Br. J. Pharmacol.* 1988;**95** (Proceedings Suppl.):770.
45 Frick WE, Sedgwick JB, Busse WW. Hypodense eosinophils in allergic rhinitis. *J. Allergy Clin. Immunol.* 1988;**82**:119–125.
46 Peters MS, Gleich GJ, Dunnette SL, Fukuda T. Ultrastructural study of eosinophils from patients with the hypereosinophilic syndrome: a morphological basis of hypodense eosinophils. *Blood* 1988;**71**:780–785.
47 Winqvist I, Olofsson T, Olsson I, Persson A–M, Hallberg T. Altered density, metabolism and surface receptors of eosinophils in eosinophilia. *Immunology* 1982;**47**:531–539.
48 Khalife J, Capron M, Grzych JM, Bazin H, Capron A. Extracellular release of rat eosinophil peroxidase (EPO). I. Role of anaphylactic immunoglobulins. *J. Immunol.* 1985;**134**:1968–1974.
49 Slifman NR, Adolphson CR, Gleich GJ. Eosinophils: biochemical and cellular aspects. In *Allergy: Principles and Practice,* 3rd edn (Eds Middleton E, Reed CE, Ellis EF, Adkinson NF, Yunginger JW), Mosby, St Louis 1988, pp. 179–205.
50 Snyderman R, Verghese MW. Leukocyte activation by chemoattractant receptors: role of guanine nucleotide regulatory protein and polyphosphoinositide metabolism. *Rev. Infect. Dis.* 1987;**9** (Suppl. 5):s562–569.
51 Ligeti E, Doussiere J, Vignais PV. Activation of the O_2-generating oxidase in plasma membrane from bovine polymorphonuclear neutrophils by arachidonic acid, a cytosolic factor of protein nature, and nonhydrolipable analogues of GTP. *Biochemistry* 1988;**27**:193–200.
52 Burgoyne RD, Cheek TR, O'Sullivan AJ. Receptor activation of phospholipase A_2 in cellular signalling. *Trends Biochem. Sci.* 1987;**12**:332–333.

11 · Eosinophil granule proteins in bronchial asthma

P. Venge and Marie Carlson

Introduction

Blood eosinophilia is one of the hallmarks of bronchial asthma. Thus, several studies have demonstrated a relationship between the extent of the blood eosinophilia and the severity of asthma [1,2]. In spite of this fact the precise role of the eosinophil in asthma has stayed enigmatic. During recent years the hypothesis has grown popular that the eosinophil might play a causative role in bronchial asthma since it has been shown that the eosinophil is a potent proinflammatory cell with the capacity to produce a number of principles of interest in this regard. These are an array of highly cytotoxic secretory proteins [3,4] and the bronchoconstrictory agents leukotriene (LT) C_4 [5,6] and platelet-activating factor (PAF) [7]. The knowledge of the biological functions of the secretory proteins has become of major importance in our understanding of the function of the eosinophil. Also the availability of sensitive immunoassays for the measurements of some of these secretory granule proteins in various body fluids such as serum, bronchoalveolar lavage fluid, sputum, etc., has provided us with unique possibilities to monitor the extent of the eosinophil involvement *in vivo* in bronchial asthma. In this chapter we will review our current knowledge of the biological functions of the eosinophil granule proteins with emphasis on their possible role in asthma and our current clinical knowledge from the measurement of the proteins.

Biochemistry and function of the human eosinophil

Morphologically the eosinophil is characterized by its abundance of eosin staining granules, which contain as major constituents some highly basic proteins. Four of these proteins have been purified and characterized in detail. These are ECP (eosinophil cationic protein) [8,9], EPO (eosinophil peroxidase) [10], EPX/EDN (eosinophil protein-X/eosinophil derived neurotoxin) [11,12] and MBP (major basic protein) [13]. With the exception of EPO, which has a molecular weight of 67 000, these proteins are fairly small with molecular weights ranging from about 10 000 to 23 000. Eosinophil cationic protein and EPX/EDN show a 40% sequence homology in the amino terminal end of the proteins, which suggests a close relationship [14]. This relationship is also indicated by the fact that one monoclonal antibody raised against ECP also reacts with an epitope on the EPX/EDN molecule [15]. Contrary to this relationship MBP seems to be a completely distinct protein [16]. By immunohistological techniques MBP has been shown to be contained within the crystalloid granules of human eosinophils and is probably the protein making up the crystal [17]. Eosinophil peroxidase and ECP are contained in the matrix of the same granules. In addition ECP has been shown to be contained within a population of small EPO-negative granules [17]. We have recently separated eosinophil granules on sucrose density gradients and measured the distribution of the three proteins ECP, EPO and EPX/EDN in the gradient [18]. These studies revealed four distinct peaks containing both ECP and EPX/EDN but of which only the heaviest peak contained EPO. The distribution of the proteins in the lightest peak coincided with the distribution of markers for plasma membranes which suggested the binding of the proteins to the plasma membrane. Thus, we concluded from these studies and from the studies related above that there is a considerable heterogeneity as to the size and density of the granules in human eosinophils, but also as to the protein content of the granules, with one very dense granule population containing EPO in addition to ECP, EPX/EDN and MBP and two less dense granule populations only containing ECP and EPX/EDN.

Release of the granule proteins from the eosinophils may be triggered by several means. Thus, large sephadex beads coated with serum proteins and probably triggering through the C3b receptor is a fairly potent stimulus for the release of ECP and EPX/EDN but not for EPO [18]. Also the triggering of the cell through the IgG Fc-receptor induced an ECP release but no release of EPO [19]. In contrast EPO and MBP were shown to be selectively released when the eosinophil was stimulated through the IgE Fc-receptor. Furthermore, the exposure of the eosinophil to the protein kinase C agonist $IpOCOC_9$, a diglyceride, induced a heavy EPX/EDN release but only moderate ECP and EPO release [18]. These data would suggest that the release of the four granule proteins from the human eosinophil is a selective process in spite of the fact that the proteins to some extent are contained within the same granule populations.

The major known biological activity of the eosinophil granule proteins is their cytotoxicity towards both mammalian and non-mammalian cells such as respiratory epithelium, nervous tissue and schistosomula of *Schistosoma mansoni* [3,4]. One suggested mechanism of action of the cytotoxicity of ECP is the capacity of this protein to make pores in cellular membranes [20], which allows for the passage of water and ions. Eosinophil peroxidase is a potent peroxidase which in the presence of H_2O_2 and halide ions inflict damage to cells by halidation of membrane molecules. Furthermore the combined action of ECP and the EPO-H_2O_2-halide system greatly potentiates the cytotoxicity of either of the two [21]. The mechanism for the cytotoxic action of EPX/EDN and MBP is not known although the potent ribonuclease activity of the former may be of considerable interest in this context [22,23]. Other biological activities of interest is the stimulation of histamine release from mast-cells and basophils by ECP (24) and MBP (14) and the fact that ECP and EPX/EDN are able to potently inhibit T-lymphocyte proliferation [25], after mitogen stimulation or in a mixed leucocyte reaction, by a non-cytotoxic mechanism. Also the newly discovered capacity of ECP to stimulate hyaluronic acid synthesis by human fibroblasts may be relevant in the discussion of the role of eosinophils in asthma [Bengt Särnstrand *et al.* to be published].

The above list of some of the potential biological activities of the eosinophil granule proteins emphasizes the potency of the cell. One of the major questions is therefore whether these proteins are present in tissues at sufficient quantities to exert these activities and whether any evidence of such activities exists. From autopsy studies of patients dying from asthma or accidentally killed the presence of large numbers of eosinophils in the asthmatic lung has long been known and in addition to eosinophil infiltration the histopathology of the lung tissue is fairly typical with basement membrane thickening in the bronchial wall, cellular aggregates in the lumen and areas with epithelial cell injuries. By instillation of small amounts of ECP into the airways of experimental animals a very similar pathology was produced, i.e. patchy destruction of the epithelial cell layer and cellular aggregates in the lumen [26]. Immunohistological examination of the airways epithelium in biopsy material from asthmatic patients showed heavy deposition of anti-ECP immunoreactive material adjacent to areas of epithelial cell layer destruction. Eosinophil cationic protein was detected as expected within the eosinophils infiltrating the bronchial wall but also found extracellularly to a large extent particularly in those areas with signs of epithelial injury [27]. These studies would support the notion that the eosinophil, by means of the release of cytotoxic material, is involved in the production of the pathology of asthma. The question, however, whether sufficient amounts of cytotoxic proteins are present to produce the damage is very difficult to answer with certainty, but in one study huge MBP concentrations were measured in sputum of asthmatic individuals [14]. We and others have measured the concentrations in bronchoalveolar lavage fluid and found raised levels [28–30], but the problems of a correct estimation from such data of the protein concentrations in the lining fluid has prevented any far reaching conclusions.

Eosinophil granule proteins in bronchial asthma

Sensitive radioimmunoassays of all four proteins have been developed which allow the measurement of the protein concentrations in various body fluids. The most studied protein in asthma so far is ECP, which has been measured both in serum, bronchoalveolar lavage fluid, sputum and nasal washings.

Eosinophil granule proteins in serum

The first study on serum levels of ECP was made on a group of asthmatics with both extrinsic and intrinsic asthma [31]. The patients had on average highly raised eosinophil counts in blood. Unexpectedly, however, the serum ECP levels were on average only somewhat increased with a group of patients even having subnormal levels. The wide variation in serum ECP levels in asthmatics was confirmed in a subsequent study and in particular seen in patients with intrinsic asthma [32]. The reason for the low levels of ECP is still unclear but most results point to a rapid elimination and consumption of ECP during active asthma as one possibility. Thus when EPX/EDN was measured in serum from patients with active asthma the levels were invariably raised [33]. The hypothesis of an accelerated elimination of ECP during certain conditions were subsequently supported by measurements of serum ECP levels after allergen inhalation challenge [34,35]. Thus under these conditions the ECP levels were almost invariably reduced after challenge to levels significantly lower than the prechallenge levels. In about one-third of the patients, however, this reduction was preceded by a rapid and transient increment of ECP during the first hour after challenge. The significantly reduced levels of ECP were still observed 6 h after challenge but in most cases replaced by a normalization or even raised levels after 24 h. Serum levels of EPX/EDN did not show any signs of a reduction after allergen challenge but in the cases with initially raised ECP levels also the EPX/EDN levels were raised.

In a recent study on exercise-induced asthma a similar reduction of the serum ECP levels was observed [Venge *et al.* to be published]. In contrast, in a control group of asthmatics, who did not react by an asthmatic reaction to exercise, no reduction in ECP was seen. Since the ECP reduction followed the immediate asthmatic reaction after allergen or exercise we also studied the effects of histamine and metacholine challenge of asthmatics to test the possibility that the ECP reduction was a simple consequence of bronchoconstriction. However, under these circumstances no significant changes in ECP levels were seen. Our conclusions from all these clinical data on serum ECP levels in asthmatics are that the levels of ECP reflect the net result of the production, i.e. the release of ECP from the eosinophils, and the elimination from the blood and that in asthma something is produced as part of the asthmatic process that enhances the elimination rate of ECP. In fact the normal elimination rate of ECP has been estimated to be about 30 min ($t_{1/2}$) and after allergen challenge about 15 min, i.e. approximately twice as fast [unpublished]. Interestingly, inhaled budesonide and to a lesser extent disodium cromoglycate appeared to inhibit the reduction in ECP levels as a consequence of both allergen and exercise challenge in contrast to the β_2-agonist, terbutaline, which was without any effect, in spite of the complete abrogation of the immediate asthmatic reaction by the latter. In fact terbutaline seemed to add to the reduction most likely due to the below mentioned inhibition of eosinophil degranulation.

Another possible contributing factor, which has emerged as a result of the above described selective release of the various eosinophil granule proteins and which has to be borne in mind, are differences in the release of the proteins from the eosinophil *in vivo* under various conditions. At present, however, this possibility does not seem very attractive since it would mean an active turning off of the ECP release as a consequence of the asthmatic reaction. Today the only means known to inhibit the release of ECP from the eosinophils is by pharmacological means such as glucocorticosteroids and β-adrenergic drugs [36]. Therefore the challenge to solve this particular question would be to identify the principles that are formed as consequences of the asthmatic reaction and which so drastically affect the ECP-levels. As part of these efforts we have identified two substances which form complexes with ECP and therefore might be operative in this regard *in vivo* since it is well known that complexes between molecules generally are eliminated much faster, due to specific elimination mechanisms, than the uncomplexed molecules. One is the 1:1 molecular complex formed between heparin and ECP [unpublished]. The other is the capacity of α_2-macroglobulin to bind ECP [37]. This latter binding seems to be unique since it involves the specific protease binding region of α_2-macroglobulin although ECP has no proteolytic capabilities. Therefore, for this binding to take place it requires a brief exposure of α_2-macroglobulin to a proteolytic enzyme such as thrombin or cathepsin G from the neutrophils. Based on these findings one speculation is that α_2-macroglobulin is exposed to proteolytic enzymes during the asthmatic reaction and that this exposure provides the requirements for the complex formation between ECP and α_2-macroglobulin to take place. Indeed several sources of proteolytic enzymes are available in the processes leading to the immediate asthmatic reaction such as the mast-cell proteases and the proteases of the coagulation cascade to mention a few.

Relation of serum ECP levels to the asthmatic disease

Horn *et al.* have earlier shown a relationship between blood eosinophilia and the severity of asthma [1,2]. Recent studies have extended these observations and demonstrated firm relationships between the reactivity of the lung in several respects and the activity of the eosinophils as measured by serum levels of eosinophil granule proteins. These include some studies which demonstrate positive correlations between serum levels of ECP and the reactivity of the lung after challenge. One study suggested that measurements of the eosinophil granule proteins ECP or EPX might be used to predict the outcome of an inhalation allergen challenge with respect to the occurrence of a late asthmatic reaction (LAR) [35]. Thus serum levels of ECP and EPX were significantly raised before challenge in those patients who reacted with a definite LAR upon challenge. However, also in the group of patients in which a late asthmatic reaction was equivocal the protein levels were significantly raised as compared with those in the patients who had a definite negative LAR. This actually suggested that serum measurements of ECP and EPX might be a more sensitive means to monitor the processes going on in the lung than the clinical monitoring of LAR. In another study ECP in serum was measured in asthmatic patients before exercise and correlated to the exercise-induced asthma (EIA) [Venge *et al.* to be published]. A highly significant linear correlation was found between the extent of EIA and serum ECP levels before exercise suggesting a relationship between the activity of the eosinophil and the hyperreactivity of the asthmatic lung. As was demonstrated after allergen inhalation challenge the ECP levels increased initially in some patients after exercise. As discussed above this increment, however, was replaced by a significant reduction of ECP at 60 min after challenge. In another group of asthmatics, which was selected because of the absence in these patients of EIA, the prechallenge levels of ECP were on average significantly lower than in the EIA group and also lower than a non-asthmatic reference population with no changes after exercise.

Another indication of a relationship between lung hyperreactivity and the activity of the eosinophils came from a study on atopic patients with seasonal symptoms [38]. In this group of patients serum ECP levels increased significantly during the pollen season. Also lung reactivity as measured by histamine PC_{20} increased during season and correlated significantly with the ECP levels. In the same study another group of seasonal allergic patients were treated by immunotherapy. In this group no changes in ECP were seen during season and this lack of change was paralleled by a reduction in lung hyperreactivity and use of medication.

Eosinophil granule proteins in bronchoalveolar lavage, sputum and nasal washings

Bronchoalveolar lavage has proved to be an invaluable tool in the definition of the processes going on in the lung for various diseases. In asthma BAL has been performed in a number of studies and demonstrated raised numbers of eosinophils in most studies but also raised numbers of neutrophils in some [28–30,39]. Counting the number does not provide us with any information as to the active participation of the cells in the disease and one means to provide such information might be to measure the levels of secretion products in the extracellular medium. In one study BAL was performed in a group of allergic asthmatics 6–7 h after allergen inhalation challenge [28]. Some of the patients reacted with a late asthmatic response to the challenge and some only had an immediate response or no response at all. In those responding with LAR the number of eosinophils were significantly higher than in the two other groups indicating an active attraction of eosinophils only in those patients who reacted with LAR. Measuring ECP in BAL fluid demonstrated a similar pattern indicating that the eosinophils had been actively secreting their granule proteins in the lung. These same patients were challenged a second time and BAL was performed this time 2–3 h after challenge, i.e. well before the development of LAR. In this situation no eosinophilia was found. However, the ECP levels showed a tendency towards higher levels which in fact were not different from the levels at 6–7 h. This suggested that the eosinophils already at this stage were involved in the process although it was not apparent from counting the number of cells. This study has been extended by a controlled trial of the effects of inhaled budesonide [Jan deMonchy *et al.* to be published]. The patients were premedicated with inhalation of 400 μg daily or placebo for 14 days before allergen challenge and BAL. In the placebo situation significantly raised levels of ECP were observed after challenge when compared with the period of budesonide inhalation. No difference, however, in the number of eosinophils was discernible indicating that this low dose of budesonide only had the capacity to turn off secretion of the eosinophils and not the mobilization to the lung. It should be pointed out that LAR was significantly inhibited as well. In this study myeloperoxidase, MPO, was measured as a sign of neutrophil involvement. The absence of any raised levels and any effects of budesonide indicated that the neutrophils were not involved in these patients.

In the pollen season study mentioned above BAL was performed in12 atopic patients before and during season [40]. Half of the patients were pretreated with immunotherapy. Before the pollen season low numbers of eosinophils were found in all patients. In spite of this the ECP levels in BAL fluid were somewhat raised in the non-treated group. During season the numbers of eosinophils rose significantly but only in the non-treated group. This was paralleled by a slight but significant elevation of ECP. These findings were contrasted by the absence of any changes in neutrophil counts and in MPO levels. The non-treated patients had significantly more symptoms than the immunotherapy-treated group. Also the development of a lung hyperreactivity as measured by PC_{20} was absent in the treated group indicating a relationship between the reactivity and the eosinophil involvement in the lung.

In studies by other raised levels of eosinophil granule proteins were found in BAL of asthmatics without challenge [29,30]. These studies also indicated a relationship between the eosinophil involvement in the lung and lung function. Furthermore huge concentrations of MBP were described in sputa of asthmatics [14], indicating that the levels we measure in BAL only represent a minor fraction of the concentrations that may be present locally in the bronchi. Gross underestimation of the eosinophil granule proteins in BAL is likely to happen due to the extreme stickiness of most of these proteins and their tendency to adsorb to almost any surface.

The obvious problems of performing repeated BAL in order to study the kinetics of the allergic process has turned the attention to the nose. Thus ECP measurements in nasal washings have demonstrated increased levels with relations to the symptoms of the individuals [41]. Also the ECP measurements after nasal allergen challenge showed greatly increased levels which were completely normalized by pretreatment with local budesonide treatment [Hans Bisgaard *et al.* to be published]. In one study nasal washings were performed almost daily during several months in a group of seasonal allergic patients [Ulf Pipkorn *et al.* to be published]. The variations in ECP levels followed closely the variations in nasal symptoms and peaked regularly about 1 week after the peak in pollen counts. This kinetics is very similar to the one observed with serum measurements of ECP as described above. The ECP peaks also showed a tendency to follow the peaks in TAME-esterase levels by some days. These data therefore suggest an interesting temporal relationship indicating that the eosinophil involvement in the process is fairly late but that this involvement is accompanied by increments in symptoms, suggesting a causal relationship.

Do asthmatic eosinophils have an increased propensity to release their granule proteins?

As part of our hypothesis of the relationship between eosinophils and asthma we have postulated that asthmatic eosinophils are primed such that they have an enhanced response to chemotactic factors from the lung. This postulate was a consequence of our attempts to explain the selective accumulation of eosinophils in the lung in asthma in spite of the fact that the signals, the chemotactic factors, produced in the lungs did not show any selectivity [40]. This postulate proved to be correct since we could show that asthmatic eosinophils in contrast to normal eosinophils responded significantly better to almost any chemotactic factor than asthmatic neutrophils [Lena Håkansson *et al.* to be published]. We therefore extended our study and asked ourselves whether also the secretory response of the asthmatic eosinophils was primed [Marie Carlson *et al.* to be published]. A mixed population of granulocytes were incubated with a standard stimulus, i.e. serum opsonized G-15 sephadex particles, and the release of ECP and MPO was measured after 0, 5 and 20 min. Cells were obtained from 30 asthmatic patients with different severities of their disease. Eighteen non-asthmatic, apparently healthy subjects were used as controls. After 5 and 20 min the release of ECP was about twice as high ($p < 0.05$ and $p = 0.001$, respectively) as the release from the eosinophils of the reference group. Also the release of MPO from the asthmatic neutrophils was somewhat higher after 20 min ($p = 0.03$). These results suggested that the eosinophils of asthmatic subjects have an increased propensity to release their granule proteins, but contrary to the results with a selective enhancement of the migratory response of the eosinophils, the asthmatic neutrophils also showed a tendency of enhanced release of their granule proteins.

Conclusion

Our present data indicate that the measurements of granule proteins of eosinophils, such as ECP, in serum are related to the inflammatory process going on in the lung in asthma and may therefore be used as a sensitive means to monitor the disease activity in bronchial asthma. Measurements of eosinophil granule proteins in BAL, sputum and nasal washings are potent research tools and have focused the attention to a possible causal role of the eosinophil in asthma and chronic rhinitis.

Acknowledgements

Parts of the studies cited in this chapter have been supported by research grants from the Swedish Medical Research Council and AB Draco, Lund, Sweden.

References

1 Horn BR, Robin ED, Theodore J, van Kessel A. Total eosinophil counts in the management of bronchial asthma. *N. Engl. J. Med.* 1975;**292**:1152.

2 Taylor KJ, Luksza AR. Peripheral blood eosinophil counts and bronchial responsiveness. *Thorax* 1987:**42**:452–456.

3 Olsson I, Venge P. The role of the eosinophil granulocyte in the inflammatory reaction. *Allergy* 1979;**34**:353–367.

4 Gleich GJ, Flavahan NA, Fujisawa T, Vanhoutte PM. The eosinophil as a mediator of damage to respiratory epithelium: A model for bronchial hyperreactivity. *J. Allergy Clin. Immunol.* 1988;**81**:776–781.

5 Shaw RJ, Cromwell O, Kay AB. Preferential generation of leukotriene C_4 by human eosinophils. *Clin. Exp. Immunol.* 1984;70:716–722.

6 Bruynzeel PLB, Kok PTM, Viëtor RJ, Verhagen J. On the optimal conditions of LTC_4 formation by human eosinophils *in vitro*. *Prostagl. Leuktr. Med.* 1986;**20**:11–16.

7 Lee TC, Lenihan DJ, Malone B, Roddy LL, Wasserman SI. Increased biosynthesis of platelet-activating factor in activated eosinophils. *J. Biol. Chem.* 1984;**259**:5526–5532.

8 Olsson I, Venge P, Spitznagel JK, Lehrer R. Arginine-rich cationic proteins of human eosinophil granules. Comparison of the constituents of eosinophilic and neutrophilic leukocytes. *Lab. Invest.* 1977;**36**:493–500.

9 Peterson CGB, Jörnvall H, Venge P. Purification and characterization of eosinophil cationic protein from normal human eosinophils. *Eur. J. Haematol.* 1988;**40**:415–423.

10 Carlsson MGCh, Peterson CGB, Venge P. Human eosinophil peroxidase: purification and characterization. *J. Immunol.* 1985;**134**:1875–1879.

11 Durack DT, Ackerman SJ, Loegering DA, Gleich GJ. Purification of human eosinophil-derived neurotoxin. *Proc. Natl. Acad. Sci. USA* 1981;**78**:5165–5169.

12 Peterson CGB, Venge P. Purification and characterization of a new cationic protein—eosinophil protein-X(EPX)—from granules of human eosinophils. *Immunology* 1983;**50**:19–26.

13 Gleich GJ, Loegering DA, Mann KG, Maldonado JE. Comparative properties of the Charcot–Leyden crystal protein and the major basic protein from human eosinophils. *J. Clin. Invest.* 1976;**57**:633–640.

14 Gleich GJ, Adolphson CR. The eosinophil leukocyte: structure and function. *Adv. Immunol.* 1986;**39**:177–253.

15 Tai P-C, Spry CJF, Peterson C, Venge P, Olsson I. Monoclonal antibodies distinguish between storage and secreted forms of eosinophil cationic protein. *Nature* 1984;**309**:182–184.

16 Ackerman SJ, Loegering DA, Venge P, Olsson I, Harley JB, Fauci AS, Gleich GJ. Distinctive cationic proteins of the human eosinophil granule: major basic protein, eosinophil cationic protein and eosinophil-derived neurotoxin. *J. Immunol.* 1983;**131**:2977–2982.

17 Egesten A, Alumets J, von Mecklenburg C, Palmegren M, Olsson I. Localization of eosinophil cationic protein, major basic protein, and eosinophil peroxidase in human eosinophils by immunoelectron microscopic technique. *J. Histochem. Cytochem.* 1986;**34**:1399–1403.

18 Peterson CGB, Garcia RC, Carlsson MGC, Venge P. Eosinophil cationic protein(ECP), eosinophil protein X(EPX) and eosinophil peroxidase (EPO): granule distribution, degranulation and characterization of released proteins. Dissertation, 1987.

19 Capron M, Capron A. The IgE receptor of human eosinophils. In *Allergy and Inflammation* (Ed. Kay AB). Academic Press, London, 1987, pp. 151–159.

20 Ding-E Young J, Peterson CGB, Venge P, Cohn ZA. Mechanism of membrane damage mediated by human eosinophil cationic protein. *Nature* 1986;**321**:613–616.

21 Yazdanbakhsh M, Tai PC, Spry CJ, Gleich GJ, Roos D. Synergism between eosinophil cationic protein and oxygen metabolites in killing of schistosomula of *Schistosoma mansoni*. *J. Immunol.* 1987;**138**:3443–3447.

22 Gleich GJ, Loegering DA, Bell MP, Checkel JL, Ackerman SJ, McKean DJ. Biochemical and functional similarities between human eosinophil-derived neurotoxin and eosinophil cationic protein: homology with ribonuclease. *Proc. Natl. Acad. Sci. USA* 1986;**83**:3146–3150.

23 Gullberg U, Widegren B, Arnason U, Egeston A, Olsson I. The cytotoxic eosinophil cationic protein (ECP) has ribonuclease activity. *Biochem. Biophys. Res. Commun.* 1986;**139**:1239–1242.
24 Bergstrand H, Lundquist B, Peterson BÅ, Peterson CGB, Venge P. Eosinophil derived cationic proteins and human leukocyte histamine release. In *Inflammation* (Eds Venge P, Lindbom A). Almqvist & Wiksell International, Stockholm, 1985, pp. 361–366.
25 Peterson CGB, Skoog V, Venge P. Human eosinophil cationic proteins (ECP and EPX) and their suppressive effects on lymphocyte proliferation. *Immunobiology* 1986;**171**:1–13.
26 Dahl R, Venge P, Fredens K. Eosinophils. In *Asthma: Basic mechanisms and Clinical Management* (Eds Barnes PJ, Rodger I, Thomson N). Academic Press, London, 1988, pp. 115–129.
27 Venge P, Peterson CGB. Eosinophil biochemistry and killing mechanisms. In *Eosinophils in Asthma* (Eds Morley J, Colditz I). Academic Press, London, 1989, pp. 163–177.
28 DeMonchy JGR, Kauffman HF, Venge P, *et al.* Bronchoalveolar eosinophilia during allergen-induced late asthmatic reactions. *Am. Rev. Respir. Dis.* 1985;**131**:373–376.
29 Kirby JG, Hargreave FE, Gleich GJ, O'Byrne PM. Bronchoalveolar cell profiles of asthmatic and non-asthmatic subjects. *Am. Rev. Resp. Dis.* 1987;**136**:379–383.
30 Wardlaw AJ, Dunnette S, Gleich GJ, Collins JV, Kay AB. Eosinophils and mast cells in bronchoalveolar lavage in subjects with mild asthma. *Am. Rev. Resp. Dis.* 1988;**137**:62–69.
31 Venge P, Zetterström O, Dahl R, Roxin L-E, Olsson I. Low levels of eosinophil cationic proteins in patients with asthma. *Lancet* 1977;**ii**:373–375.
32 Dahl R, Venge P. Role of the eosinophil in bronchial asthma. In *Corticosteroid Treatment in Allergic Airway Diseases* (Eds Clark TJH, Mygind N, Selroos O), Munksgaard, Copenhagen, 1982, pp. 23–28.
33 Venge P, Dahl R, Fredens K, Hällgren R, Peterson C. Eosinophil cationic proteins (ECP and EPX) in health and disease. In *Immunobiology of the Eosinophil* (Eds Yoshida T, Torisu M), Elsevier Science, New York. 1983, pp. 163–179.
34 Dahl R, Venge P, Olsson I. Variations of blood eosinophils and cationic protein in serum in patients with bronchial asthma. Studies during inhalation challenge test. *Allergy* 1978;**33**:211–215.
35 Venge P, Dahl R, Peterson CGB. Eosinophil granule proteins in serum after allergen challenge of asthmatic patients and the effects of anti-asthmatic medication. *Int. Arch. Allergy Appl. Immun.* 1988;**87**:306–312.
36 Dahl R, Venge P. Blood eosinophil count and eosinophil cationic protein. *In vivo* study of the influence of beta-2-adrenergic drugs and steroid medication. *Scand. J. Resp. Dis.* 1978;**59**:319–322.
37 Peterson CGB, Venge P. Interaction and complex formation between the eosinophil cationic protein (ECP) and alpha-2-macroglobulin. *Biochem. J.* 1987;**245**:781–787.
38 Rak S, Löwhagen O, Venge P. The effect of immunotherapy on bronchial hyperresponsiveness and eosinophil cationic protein in pollen allergic patients. *J. Allergy Clin. Immunol.* 1988;**82**:470–480.
39 Metzger WJ, Richerson HB, Worden K, Monick M, Hunninghake G. Bronchoalveolar lavage in allergic asthmatic patients following allergen provocation. *Chest* 1986;**89**:477.
40 Rak S, Björnsson A, Håkansson L, Sörenson S, Venge P. Immunotherapy prevents eosinophil accumulation and production of eosinophil chemotactic activity in the lung of asthmatics during natural allergen challenge. Dissertation, 1988.
41 Linder A, Venge P, Deuschl H. Eosinophil cationic protein and myeloperoxidase in nasal secretion as makers of inflammation in allergic rhinitis. *Allergy* 1987;**42**:583–590.

12 · Mononuclear cell-derived eosinophil-activating factors

Kareen J.I. Thorne, B.A. Richardson and A.E. Butterworth

Eosinophils from different donors differ widely in their cytotoxic activities. Populations of eosinophils of different densities have been isolated from the blood of different donors: moderately eosinophilic donors have eosinophils which sediment on centrifuging in a metrizamide gradient to the 23/24% metrizamide interface [1], hypereosinophilic syndrome patients produce in addition eosinophils of light density which sediment to the 18/20 and 20/22% interfaces [2]. Within the population of normal density eosinophils a wide-range of cytotoxic activities have been observed. Cytotoxic activity may be measured from the ability of eosinophils to mediate antibody-dependent killing of schistosomula of *Schistosoma mansoni*. Some correlation has been observed between cytotoxic activity and blood eosinophilia [3].

Mononuclear cells from individuals with high activity eosinophils secrete substances which enhance the cytotoxic activity of low activity eosinophils [4,5]. Mononuclear cells are incubated for 16 h in tissue culture medium containing either fetal calf serum, or bovine serum albumin, but without further stimulus. The cell free supernatant is collected and tested for its ability to enhance the cytotoxic activity of low activity eosinophils. Mononuclear cell supernatants from an eosinophilic donor enhance antibody-dependent, and to a limited extent antibody-independent, killing of schistosomula. Normal donors do not produce this eosinophil-activating activity. The activity appears to reside in protein as it is lost after trypsin treatment.

Mononuclear cell supernatants appear to contain a number of different components with eosinophil-activating activity. After separation by isoelectric focusing several peaks of activity are found, all with acidic pIs. Gel filtration shows the presence of components of molecular weights > 100, 40 and < 10 kD. Several proteins with eosinophil-activating activity have now been purified from mononuclear cell supernatants and characterized (Tables 12.1 and 12.2). Eosinophil activating factor (EAF) is the main product from mononuclear cells incubated without further stimulation. Tumour necrosis factor (TNF) is formed when monocytes are treated with LPS. Monocyte-derived eosinophil cytotoxicity enhancing factor (M-ECEF) probably contains TNF and EAF and possibly also the 10 kD factor. The 10 kD protein is produced by U937 cells and by blood monocytes after treatment with PMA and LPS. Certain human colony stimulating factors also increase the cytotoxic activity of human blood eosinophils. These include a factor from eosinophilic serum which is an eosinophil colony stimulating factor, the eosinophil CSF interleukin-5 (IL-5),

Table 12.1. Factors from human mononuclear cells which enhance the cytotoxic activity of eosinophils

Factor	Source	Reference no.
EAF	Monocytes from eosinophilic donors	4–7
M-ECEF	Monocytes+LPS; U937+PMA+LPS	17–19
TNF*	Monocytes+LPS	20
10 K factor	U937+PMA+LPS	21

*Enhanced by γ-interferon.

Table 12.2. Human colony stimulating factors which enhance the cytotoxic activity of eosinophils

Factor	Source	CSF	Reference no.
Serum factor (80 kD)	Eosinophilic serum; T-cell clones	Eo	8,9
IL-5	Recombinant	Eo	22
GM-CSF	Monocytes; T-cells	Eo,N,M	23
IL-3	T-cells	Pluripotent	24

granulocyte macrophage-colony stimulating factor (GM-CSF) and the pluripotent CSF IL-3. Factors which do not enhance the cytotoxic activity of eosinophils include α-interferon (IFN), γ-IFN, IL-1, IL-2, G-CSF and M-CSF. γ-IFN does however have a synergistic effect on eosinophil activation by TNF. It does not have an effect on eosinophil activation by EAF.

We will concentrate in the rest of this paper on the EAF. This can be partially purified from mononuclear cell supernatants by gel filtration on Sephacryl-S200, followed by ion-exchange chromatography on DEAE [6]. It can be separated from CSFs and from TNF activity by HPLC on DEAE-5PW [7]. Silver stained SDS-PAGE reveals the presence of one major protein and several minor ones in the active fractions; these are in the 50 kD region. On gel filtration EAF appears to have a molecular weight of about 40 kD. Evidence has been obtained that EAF is a glycoprotein. It binds to the lectin-agaroses glycosylex and agarose ricinus, but does not bind to fucosylex. Production of EAF in the presence of tunicamycin to inhibit glycosylation modifies the elution pattern during HPLC on DEAE-5PW.

Formation of EAF occurs in both monocytes and lymphocytes. When crude cell supernatants are analysed for eosinophil activating activity only monocytes, and not lymphocytes, appear to be active producers. After purification, however, eosinophil activating activity is found from both monocytes and lymphocytes (Fig. 12.1). Lymphocyte EAF is liberated from its latent state during the gel filtration stage of purification. Dialysis does not activate it.

Table 12.3. Immunological properties of eosinophils in different state of activation

	Normal density		
	−EAF	+EAF	Light density
Cell-mediated cytotoxicity			
Ab independent	0	0/+	0
IgG dependent	++	+++	0
IgE dependent	0	0	++
Adherence			
Ab independent	0	0/+	0
IgG dependent	++	+++	++
IgE dependent	+	++	++
Surface receptors			
FcεRII (BB10)	0	?	++
CR3 a-chain (CD11b)	+	++	++

Recent work by Dr Jamal Khalife has shown that an eosinophilic activating activity can be detected in serum from eosinophilic donors. Investigations are in progress to discover if this activity is due to EAF in serum, or possibly to the eosinophil CSF discovered by Dr Peter Kern [8,9].

We have developed a human cell line, ESH 98, as an alternative source of EAF [10]. This cell line was formed by fusing human cervical keratinocytes with HeLa cells. It can be induced to secrete eosinophil activating activity by stimulation with TNF. The activity co-purifies with EAF. It has similar biochemical and morphological effects on eosinophils to the effects observed with mononuclear cell EAF.

The effects of mononuclear cell EAF on eosinophils have been investigated in some detail. EAF-activated eosinophils differ from the light density eosinophils isolated from HES patients (immunological properties are shown in Table 12.3). EAF

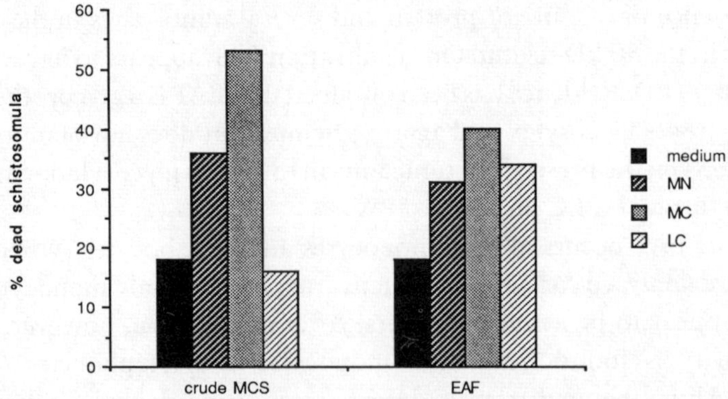

Fig. 12.1. Production of EAF by blood monocytes and lymphocytes.

enhances IgG-mediated cytotoxic activity, light density eosinophils exhibit IgE-mediated cytotoxicity; EAF enhances adherence to IgG and to IgE coated targets, light density eosinophils have FcεRII receptors; EAF-activated and light density eosinophils both exhibit CR3 receptors for C3bi [11]. EAF has marked effects on the release of cytotoxic proteins from eosinophils. While the total content of cytotoxic proteins does not change markedly, the proportion of cells staining positively with EG2, a monoclonal antibody which recognizes only the secreted form and not the storage form of ECP, is increased both in EAF-activated and in light density eosinophils [12]. Eosinophil peroxidase secretion is increased in EAF-activated cells either without further stimulation or in the presence of opsonized zymosan, but is increased in light density eosinophils only in response to specific antigen or anti-IgE. Eosinophil-activating factor-activated cells differ from light density cells in enhanced production of superoxide and hydrogen peroxide and increased NBT reduction [7]. Leukotriene (LT) C_4 production, induced by IgG beads is enhanced by EAF, but is greater in light density cells [13].

Eosinophil-activating factor induces marked morphological changes in the eosinophil. Nomarski optics reveal that the cell is changed from small and spherical to large and flattened. These changes have been examined in more detail by electron microscopy. During 2 h of incubation with EAF the cell changes shape and sends out lamellipodia [14]. Eosinophil activating factor need only be present for 2 h for the cells to be fully activated and to retain their activity over a subsequent 40 h incubation with schistosomula. The distribution of polymerized actin was investigated with NBD-phallacidin. A change in distribution from evenly over the whole cell to localization in the lamellipodia was observed [10]. It has been shown that cells activated with

Table 12.4. Effects of EAF on eosinophils

Enhances IgG mediated cytotoxicity
Enhances IgG mediated adherence
Enhances expression of receptor for C3bi
Converts ECP from stored to secreted form
Increases secretion of ECP
Increases secretion of EPO
Increases production of superoxide
Increases production of hydrogen peroxide
Increases reduction of nitroblue tetrazolium
Increases secretion of LTC_4
Increases uptake of deoxyglucose
Changes cell surface proteins
Induces changes in cell morphology

mononuclear cell supernatants also change their surface properties; a panel of monoclonal antibodies to the eosinophil surface was used to detect changes [15].

Effects of EAF on eosinophils are summarized in Table 12.4: it enhances cytotoxic properties of eosinophils; increases secretion of cytotoxic proteins, toxic oxygen metabolities and LTC_4; induces changes in the morphology of the eosinophil. TNF resembles EAF in some of its properties: it enhances IgG-mediated cytotoxicity, increases LTC_4 production, enhances CR3 expression and has no colony stimulating nor chemotactic activity. A colony stimulating factor which also prolongs cell survival is GM-CSF: it enhances cytotoxicity, increases phagocytosis, causes changes in cell morphology with reduced cell density and enhances superoxide production, LTC_4 production and CR3 expression. The pluripotent CSF IL-3 also enhances superoxide production and increases cytotoxic activity.

In an evaluation of the pathological significance of EAF we have measured the production of EAF by blood monocytes obtained from blood from patients with asthma. While cells from some patients secrete high levels of EAF a few patients secrete little or no EAF (Fig. 12.2). No correlation was found between level of EAF production and extent of eosinophilia. The effects of some of the drugs used by these patients is shown in Table 12.5. Methyl prednisolone, beclomethasone and theophylline inhibit production of EAF by mononuclear cells, while cromoglycate and salbutamol have no effect. None of the drugs tested affected eosinophil activation by EAF in our assays [16].

A possible role for cytokines in EAF formation was investigated. Although some

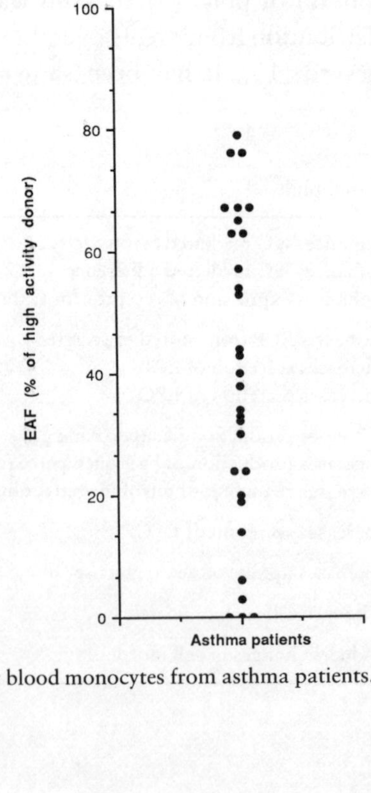

Fig. 12.2. Production of EAF by blood monocytes from asthma patients.

enhancement of the production of eosinophil activating activity was observed when mononuclear cells were incubated with IL 1–5 or with IL-2, this activity was not due to EAF and could be ascribed, at least in part, to TNF.

Allergens do appear to play a role in the induction of EAF formation. In Table 12.6 are shown the responses of four individuals to different allergens. Production of EAF was enhanced in different individuals by different allergens. Extracts of *Dermatophagoides pteronyssinus*, *Candida albicans* and ragweed pollen (100 μg/ml) all proved effective in certain individuals. Lymphocyte proliferation in response to these allergens was also measured.

The important areas for further work appear to be the relative roles of the lymphocyte and the monocyte, the activation of these cells by different allergens and the significance of the latency of the activity produced by lymphocytes.

Table 12.5. Inhibitors of EAF production by mononuclear cells

Inhibited by:	
methyl prednisolone	0.1 μg/ml
beclomethasone	0.1–1 μg/ml
theophylline	100 μg/ml
Not inhibited by:	
cromoglycate (intal)	100 μg/ml
salbutamol (ventolin)	100 μg/ml

None of the above drugs inhibit eosinophil activation by EAF.

Table 12.6. Response of blood mononuclear cells to allergens

	EAF production (% dead schistosomula)				Cell proliferation (^{3}H thymidine incorporation)			
	A	B	C	D	A	B	C	D
Medium	20	4	23	20	600	700	5000	1600
D. pteronyssinus	32	29	31	—	5000	32750	10000	—
C. albicans	39	39	23	26	45000	92000	71000	6000
Rye grass	17	19	27	25	600	1800	25000	3000
Ragweed	18	7	22	30	700	—	21000	1900
Unstimulated eosinophils	3	3	15	15				

References

1 Vadas MA, David JR, Butterworth A, Pisani NT, Siongok TA. A new method for the purification of human eosinophils, and a comparison of the ability of these cells to damage schistosomula of *Schistosoma mansoni*. *J. Immunol.* 1979;**122**:1228.

2 Prin L, Capron M, Tonnel AB, Bletry O, Capron A. Heterogeneity of human peripheral blood eosinophils: variability in cell density and cytotoxic ability in relation to the level and origin of hypereosinophilia. *Int. Arch. Allergy Appl. Immunol.* 1983;**72**:336.

3 David JR, Vadas MA, Butterworth AE, Azevedo de Brito P, Carvalho EM, David RA, Bina JC, Andrade ZA. Enhanced helminthotoxic capacity of eosinophils from patients with eosinophilia. *N. Engl. J. Med.* 1980;**303**:1147.

4 Veith MC, Butterworth AE. Enhancement of human eosinophil-mediated killing of *Schistosoma mansoni* larvae by mononuclear cell products *in vitro*. *J. Exp. Med.* 1983;**157**:1828.

5 Veith MC, Taylor DW, Thorne K, Richardson BA, Butterworth AE. Studies on the enhancement of eosinophil function by mononuclear cell products *in vitro*. *Clin. Exp. Immunol.* 1984;**58**:603.

6 Thorne KJI, Richardson BA, Veith MC, Tai PC, Spry CJF, Butterworth AE. Partial purification and biological properties of an eosinophil-activating factor. *Eur. J. Immunol.* 1985;**15**:1083.

7 Thorne KJI, Richardson BA, Taverne J, Williamson DJ, Vadas MA, Butterworth AE. A comparison of eosinophil-activating factor (EAF) with other monokines and lymphokines. *Eur. J. Immunol.* 1986;**16**:1143.

8 Kern P, Dietrich M. Eosinophil differentiating activity in sera of patients with AIDS under recombinant Il-2 substitution. *Blut* 1986;**52**:249.

9 Kern P, Horstmann RD, Dietrich M. Eosinophil production in human bone-marrow cultures induced by 80–85 kDa serum component(s) of patients with eosinophilia. *Br. J. Haematol.* 1987;**66**:165.

10 Thorne KJI, Richardson BA, Butterworth AE, Stanley M. Eosinophil-activating factor (EAF) production by a human cell line (ESH98) stimulated with tumour necrosis factor. *Immunol.* 1988;**63**:545.

11 Capron M, Kazatchkine MD, Fischer E, Joseph M, Butterworth AE, Kusnierz JP, Prin L, Papin JP, Capron A. Functional role of the α-chain of complement receptor type 3 in human eosinophil-dependent antibody-mediated cytotoxicity against schistosomes. *J. Immunol.* 1987;**139**:2059.

12 Tai PC, Spry CJF, Peterson C, Venge P, Olsson I. Monoclonal antibodies distinguish between storage and secreted forms of eosinophil cationic protein. *Nature* 1984;**309**,182.

13 Fitzharris P, Moqbel R, Thorne KJI, Richardson BA, Hartnell A, Cromwell O, Butterworth AE, Kay AB. The effects of eosinophil activating factor on IgG-dependent sulphidopeptide leukotriene generation by human eosinophils. *Clin. Exp. Immunol.* 1986;**66**:673.

14 Butterworth AE, Thorne KJI. Eosinophils in parasitic diseases: properties of an eosinophil activating factor (EAF). *Eos. Riv. Immunol. Immunofarm.* 1988;8:33.

15 Tai PC, Bakes DM, Barkans JR, Spry CJF. Eosinophil membrane antigens: phenotypic frequencies in normal individuals and patients with the hypereosinophilic syndrome. *Clin. Exp. Immunol.* 1985;**60**:427.

16 Thorne KJI, Richardson BA, Butterworth AE, Hay I, Higenbottam, TW. Effect of drugs used in the treatment of asthma on the production of eosinophil-activating factor by monocytes. *Int. Arch. Allergy Appl. Immun.* 1988;**85**:257.

17 Dessein AJ, Lenzi HL, David JR. Modulation of the cytotoxicity of human blood eosinophils by factors secreted by monocytes and T lymphocytes. *Monogr. Allergy* 1983;**18**:45.

18 Dessein AJ, Lenzi HL, Bina JC, Carvalho EM, Weiser WY, Andrade ZA, David JR. Modulation of eosinophil cytotoxicity of blood mononuclear cells from healthy subjects and patients with chronic *Schistosoma mansoni*. *Cell Immunol.* 1984;**85**:100.

19 Silberstein DS, Dessein AJ, Elsas PP, Fontaine B, David JR. Characterization of a factor from the U937 cell line that enhances the toxicity of human eosinophils to *Schistosoma mansoni* larvae. *J. Immunol.* 1987;**138**:3042.

20 Silberstein DS, David JR. Tumour necrosis factor enhances eosinophil toxicity to *Schistosoma mansoni* larvae. *Proc. Natl. Acad. Sci. USA* 1986;**83**:1055.

21 Silberstein DS, David JR. The regulation of human eosinophil function by cytokines. *Immunol. Today* 1987;**8**:380.

22 Lopez AF, Sanderson CJ, Gamble JR, Campbell HD, Young IG, Vadas MA. Recombinant human interleukin 5 is a selective activator of human eosinophil function. *J. Exp. Med.* 1988;**167**:219.

23 Vadas MA, Nicola NA, Metcalf D. Activation of antibody-dependent cell-mediated cytotoxicity of human neutrophils and eosinophils by separate colony-stimulating factors. *J. Immunol.* 1983;**130**:795.

24 Rothenburg ME, Owen WF, Silberstein DS, Woods J, Soberman RJ, Austen KF, Stevens RL. Human eosinophils have prolonged survival, enhanced functional properties and become hypodense when exposed to human interleukin 3. *J. Clin. Invest.* 1988;**81**:1986.

13 · Inhibition of allergen-induced cutaneous eosinophilia by anti-allergic drugs

Christine De Vos

Introduction

The IgE-mediated mechanisms leading to mast-cell degranulation and rapid release of mediators probably account almost entirely for the clinical manifestations of immediate hypersensitivity: rhinorrhoea, blocked nose, sneezing, wheezing, pruritus, abdominal discomfort, and diarrhoea. With a single exposure to an allergen, these symptoms are self-limiting and usually subside spontaneously. However, in most models of allergenic challenge, the immediate reaction is followed by a late-phase reaction. The late reaction is associated with the migration of inflammatory cells to the site of the immediate reaction [1]. This becomes the predominant feature in the case of repeated or continued exposure to allergen.

Today allergy may be considered as a chronic disease, progressing from an acute state to a chronic condition. The study of the late-phase reaction, the association between inflammation and the allergic response and the modifications induced by these events all help in unravelling the complex mechanisms involved.

The cutaneous domain is obviously easier to investigate in man. The early and late cutaneous reactions in normal and atopic subjects have been assessed by different techniques.

Usually, the cutaneous cellular infiltration can be evaluated either by the technique of the Rebuck window [2], which is easy to perform, or by histology of a skin biopsy, which is a more difficult and also a more invasive technique. Another, more sophisticated technique is that of suction-induced blisters, followed by deroofing and the positioning of skin chambers [3]. The latter technique permits measurement, in the chamber fluid, of the concentration of the mediators which are released once the allergic reaction has been triggered, as well as investigation of the cellular infiltration.

Hallmarks of the allergic cutaneous inflammation

Inflammatory reactions are generally characterized by cellular infiltrations consisting predominantly of neutrophils, followed by monocytic leucocytes [4]. Figures 13.1 and 13.2 summarize the cellular events in a skin window stimulated by the application of ragweed allergen (Fig. 13.2) as compared with the ones occurring in a control site to which tetanus toxoid had been applied in one allergic subject (Fig. 13.1). The control site was characterized initially by the accumulation of polymorphonuclear leucocytes,

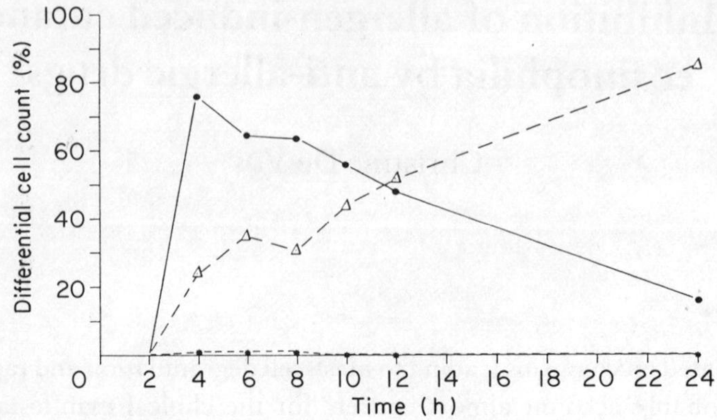

Fig. 13.1. Skin cellular recruitment in an allergic patient—Control site—Skin window technique—Application of tetanus toxoid on abraded skin. (●—●) Neutrophils, (△---△) monocytes, (*---*) eosinophils. (Reproduced from Eidinger *et al. J. Allergy* 1964;35:77–85.)

with mononuclear cells in the minority. Subsequently, however, the infiltration with polymorphonuclear leucocytes diminished whereas the mononuclear cells accumulated strikingly, so that at 24 h the infiltrate consisted mainly of mononuclear cells (Fig. 13.1). Eosinophils were occasionally noted in the early stages of the skin window response. The allergic site was, in contrast, characterized by the accumulation of eosinophils, often being the predominant cell type at the 24-h period (Fig. 13.2). This can be partly explained by the fact that, during the immediate response, some of the mediators released are chemotactic and can thus attract these leucocytes [1,5,6].

Allergen can also directly activate eosinophils, monocytes and platelets via reaction with IgE fixed to low affinity FcεII receptors. This reaction releases additional

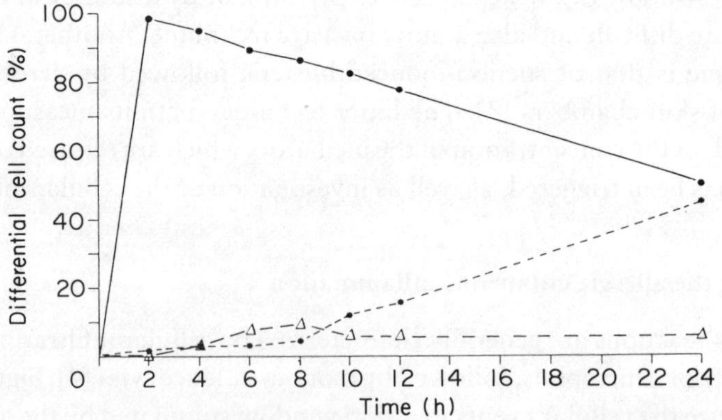

Fig. 13.2. Skin cellular recruitment in an allergic patient—Ragweed test site—Skin window technique—Application of ragweed extract on abraded skin. Symbols as in Fig. 13.1. (Reproduced from Eidinger *et al. J. Allergy* 1964;35:77–85.)

chemotactic mediators [7]. The two determinant factors that appear to be required to provoke the migration of eosinophils are first the triggering of a reaction which will release at least one factor chemotactic for eosinophils, and second the presence of atopy. These facts are supported by the work of Bryant and Kay showing in 1977 [8] that in atopic and non-atopic individuals with similar blood eosinophil counts, topical application of ECF-A tetrapeptide to the abraded skin would provoke, 24 h later, the selective migration of eosinophils only in the atopic patients; this migration was always less than that obtained after application of an allergen.

Fadel *et al.* [9] clearly established that, in healthy subjects, the cellular migration induced by histamine is no different from the one provoked by the control medium. That is to say that no eosinophils have been found under these conditions. Similarly, in allergic subjects stimulated by either the control medium or by histamine, there was no migration of eosinophils.

More recently, Henocq and Vargaftig [10] have studied the response of atopic and non-atopic volunteers to an intradermal injection of platelet activating factor (PAF)-acether or of the leucocyte secretagogue and chemoattractant formyl-methionyl-leucyl-phenylalanine (FMLP). Immediate weal and flare skin reactions were of equal intensity in both groups of subjects. The cellular responses, assessed by the Rebuck skin window technique, demonstrated a late (24 h) eosinophilic response to both inflammatory agents, with 33–44% of intensely degranulated eosinophils in atopic subjects. In comparison, very few if any eosinophils were observed in the non-atopic subjects (Fig. 13.3).

The accumulation of eosinophils in human skin indicates a potent eosinophilotactic activity restricted to the allergic patients, and which is the hallmark of the cutaneous inflammation linked to allergic triggering.

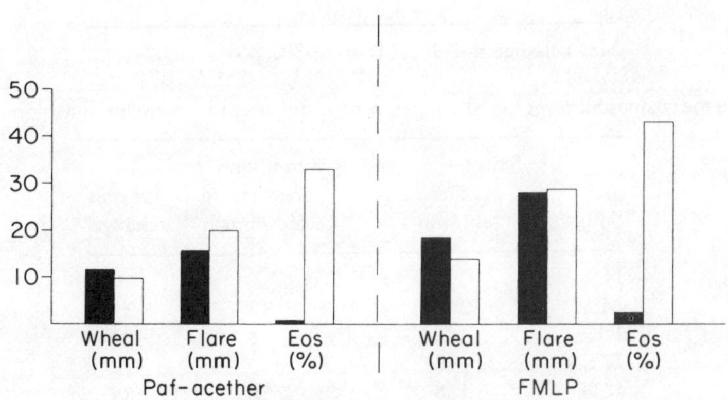

Fig. 13.3. Skin cellular recruitment in six normal (■) and six atopic subjects (□) induced by either 200 ng PAF-acether/site or 5 μg FMLP/site—Skin window technique on abraded skin. (Reproduced from Hénocq and Vargaftig *J. Allergy Clin. Immunol.* 1988;**81**:691–695.)

T-lymphocyte activation, assessed in biopsies by immunocytochemistry using a panel of monoclonal antibodies, is strongly correlated with an eosinophil activation 24 h after allergic challenge ($r = 0.94, p < 0.001$) [11]. Thus, interactions between T-lymphocytes, mast-cells and eosinophils in reactions to airborne allergens may be important, leading to an inflammation which is characteristic of the allergic response.

Pharmacological modulation of allergic cutaneous cellular infiltration

Corticosteroids do not prevent allergen-induced weal and flare reactions [12–14]. However, these substances are capable of inhibiting the inflammatory migration of cells associated with the allergic skin response.

Table 13.1 summarizes the results obtained by Dunsky *et al.* [14], who showed by biopsy that a single intravenous injection of methylprednisolone (1 mg/kg) significantly inhibited the eosinophil infiltration 2 h after allergic challenge.

As with corticosteroids, local administration of cromolyn did not modulate the ragweed-induced skin-weal response [15]. Nevertheless, in contrast to corticosteroids, cromolyn did not inhibit the recruitment of eosinophils at the skin sites challenged by ragweed allergen (Fig. 13.4).

Table 13.1a. Tissue eosinophil response to antigen before and after giving a placebo i.v.

Subject	Skin-test no. 1: pre-placebo (eos/mm^2)	Skin-test no. 3: post-placebo (eos/mm^2)	Per cent change
N.S.	32	36	+11
M.M.	74	143	+93
F.K.	84	29	−67
W.S.	217	60	−72
D.H.	51	46	−9

Mean change = −9%, SD = ±67%, $p = > 0.1$.

Table 13.1b. Tissue eosinophil response to antigen before and after i.v. methylprednisolone (1 mg/kg)

Subject	Skin-test no. 1: pre-steroid (eos/mm^2)	Skin-test no. 3: post-steroid (eos/mm^2)	Per cent change
N.S.	78	0	−100
M.M.	212	11	−94
F.K.	108	6	−94
W.S.	440	15	−96
D.H.	138	16	−88

Mean change = −94%, SD = ±4, $p = < 0.05$.

From Dunsky *et al. J. Allergy Clin. Immunol.* 1977;59:142–146.

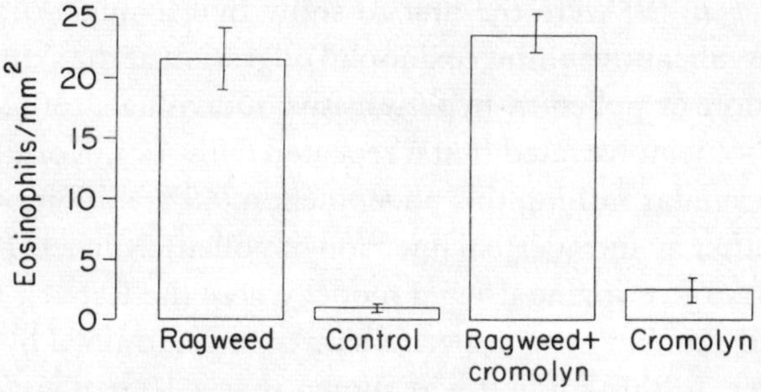

Fig. 13.4. Tissue eosinophil response (cells/mm^2) at skin sites injected 2 h earlier with ragweed, PBS, ragweed plus cromolyn, and cromolyn alone. Ragweed and ragweed-plus-cromolyn mixture induced a prominent eosinophil response, significantly greater than that induced by PBS (control), or by cromolyn alone ($n = 5$). (Reproduced from Ting *et al. J. Allergy Clin. Immunol.* 1983;71:12–17.)

Local administration of terbutaline induced a significant dose-dependent suppression of the antigen-provoked skin-weal response. Concurrently, eosinophil infiltration due to allergic challenge was inhibited by terbutaline in local administration [16] (Fig. 13.5).

Inhibition of eosinophil recruitment is a property not previously observed with H_1 antagonists. Indeed, promethazine (50 mg, four times per day) did not inhibit the influx of eosinophils after an allergic skin challenge [17].

In the new generation of non-sedating anti-H_1 compounds, cetirizine given *per os* has been reported to inhibit allergic cutaneous eosinophilic infiltration in atopic subjects [9,18,19]. Like other anti-H_1 compounds, cetirizine will also clearly inhibit the weal and flare skin reaction to histamine, to the compound 48/80 or to an allergen [18].

It should be pointed out that cetirizine will inhibit the specific cutaneous migration of eosinophils, independent of both the dose administered and the duration of the

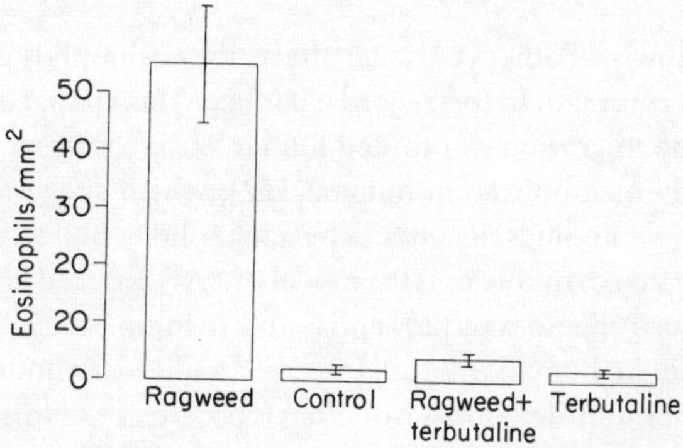

Fig. 13.5. Number of eosinophils/mm^2 accumulated on membrane filters placed 2 h earlier on blister bases which had been exposed during the previous 30 min to ragweed extract, a control solution, ragweed plus terbutaline, or terbutaline alone ($n = 5$). (From Ting *et al. J. Allergy Clin. Immunol.* 1983;71:437–441.)

treatment. Fadel *et al.* [9] were the first to show that a single oral dose of 10 mg cetirizine would significantly inhibit eosinophil migration at the skin site, 24 h after an intradermal injection of pollen in hypersensitive individuals (60% inhibition). The same team [20] also demonstrated that a repeated daily 10 mg oral dose of cetirizine would inhibit in a similar fashion this phenomenon (69% inhibition at 4 h and 62% inhibition at 24 h after an intradermal injection of pollen). Michel *et al.* [18] have confirmed this property of cetirizine using a model where the Rebuck window is placed not on the abraded skin but onto a specific skin area determined by producing a suction-induced blister. In this study it was shown that a 10 mg/day dose significantly inhibited the migration of eosinophils (65–84% inhibition at 24 h). Finally, Charlesworth *et al.* [19], using the suction-induced blister technique together with a cutaneous chamber, showed that 20 mg/day of cetirizine significantly inhibited the amount of cellular infiltrate produced by the allergic stimulus: they recorded a 65–83% inhibition of eosinophils appearing in the liquid of the chamber (see Table 13.2).

Table 13.2. Inhibition of the eosinophil recruitment by cetirizine in an allergic skin response

Authors	Reference no.	Dose of cetirizine oral route	% inhibition	Technique used
Fadel *et al.* (1987)	9	10 mg single intake	60	Dermabrasion + Rebuck window
Fadel *et al.* (1988)	20	10 mg/day	62–69	Dermabrasion + Rebuck window
Michel *et al.* (1988)	18	10 mg/day	65–84	Suction-blister + skin chamber + Rebuck window
Charlesworth *et al.* (1989)	19	20 mg/day	65–83	Suction-blister + skin chamber + cell count in the chamber fluid

It is not yet known whether cetirizine affects the eosinophils directly or rather the process of their recruitment. In this regard it has been shown that cetirizine (0.1 μg/ml) *in vitro* inhibits the migration of purified human eosinophils to PAF or FMLP [21]. Cetirizine is poorly metabolized in humans [22], which suggests that these *in vitro* data are relevant to findings *in vivo*. The ginkgolide, BN 52021, a specific PAF antagonist, is very active in this *in vitro* model of PAF-induced chemotaxis but not at all on FMLP-induced chemotaxis [23] and is able to inhibit the PAF-induced weal and flare skin reaction in humans [24]. However, sodium cromoglycate, nedocromil sodium, salbutamol and dexamethasone have no effect on this *in vitro* eosinophil PAF-induced chemotactic model [25].

All these pharmacological investigations confirm the complexity of the inflammatory skin reaction linked to the allergenic response.

Pharmacological modulation of mediator release in an allergic response

In vivo studies using the suction-blister technique have shown that neither sodium cromoglycate nor verapamil will inhibit the weal and flare reaction or the immediate release of histamine after local administration [15,26]. In contrast, terbutaline applied locally and hydroxyzine given orally, both inhibit the immediate release of histamine [16,27].

More recently [28–30], it has been shown that the amount of histamine released depends on the sensitivity of the subject and also on the duration of the contact between skin and allergen. This has also been shown by Michel *et al.* [31], using a model of a skin chamber maintained on the denuded dermis for 24 h, and which contained allergen during the first 6 h. Protein exudation and histamine assessment were followed over time. The technique itself will provoke a local reaction in both healthy and sensitized subjects. Vascular permeability increased and histamine was found in the chamber fluid during the first half-hour. Both protein exudate and histamine release were found to have decreased at 6 h, and again at 24 h. The addition of pollen to the chamber of the healthy subjects did not appear to modify these findings. In the sensitized subject, however, the reaction to allergen provoked an immediate, slight increase in protein extravasation and an increase of histamine release into the migration chamber during the first half-hour. After 6 h, an increase in protein extravasation was still noted in response to allergen stimulation and there was a sustained release of histamine. The pollen which was present in the chamber from time 0 to 6 h, was still able after 24 h to induce the late appearance of proteins and of histamine in the migration chamber, even though it was itself no longer present (Figs 13.6 and 13.7). These results, together with those produced by Atkins *et al.* [28] and Shalit *et al.* [29,30], demonstrate that maintaining pollen in the chamber for several hours produced a release of histamine which peaked within the first hour before reaching a plateau. When pollen was left in the chamber for only 1 h, the early histamine peak was not followed by a sustained plateau of production.

One interpretation of these findings, proposed by the authors, is that during prolonged exposure to the allergen—a situation which more closely resembles the clinical situation than does sudden provocation—the initial stage of mast-cell degranulation is followed by a basophil infiltration.

An oral treatment of 2×10 mg cetirizine given daily for 4 days, completely inhibited this sustained production of protein and histamine in allergic subjects (Figs 13.6 and 13.7).

Cetirizine, probably by fixing itself onto the vascular H_1-receptors, inhibited the immediate extravasation of proteins provoked by adding pollen in the chamber. On the other hand, the immediate release of histamine was not affected by the treatment, showing that, *in vivo*, cetirizine probably had no direct effect on degranulation of the mast-cells in the early phase of the allergic reaction. Nevertheless, it should be pointed

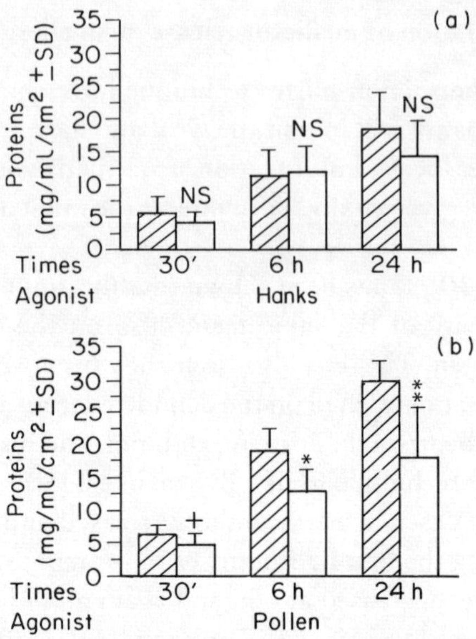

Fig. 13.6. Skin chamber technique in eight pollen-sensitive subjects. Measurement of protein diffusion into the skin chamber fluid during a specific allergic response. (a) Control situation: chambers were filled with Hank's medium (1 ml/chamber) all the time. (b) Allergic challenge: chambers were filled with pollen extract (0.01 IR/ml Hanks/chamber) from time 0 until time 6 h, and with Hank's medium (1 ml/chamber) from time 6 h until time 24 h. (▨) Placebo, (□) cetirizine 10 mg b.i.d., NS = $p > 0.1$, + = $0.05 \leqslant p \leqslant 0.1$, * = $0.01 \leqslant p \leqslant 0.05$, ** = $0.001 \leqslant p \leqslant 0.01$.

out that cetirizine inhibited the late-onset phase of protein exudation and histamine release. This action could be due to direct modification by cetirizine of either basophil or eosinophil recruitment, the latter phenomenon leading to sustained histamine release. This is, of course, one interpretation of the findings which will require further investigation to be confirmed.

Conclusion

The pathophysiological concept of allergy has developed greatly over the past few years. Not long ago, degranulation of the mast-cells, with the immediate reaction this provoked, was considered to be the key event in an allergic response. Today the complexity of the late-phase reactions occurring in the skin, the nose, the eyes and the lungs, and the changes that these pathophysiological events can cause, are considered as major events. The clinical implications of these events, i.e. bronchial hyperreactivity in the asthmatic allergic patient, shed some light on its relevance in the daily life of the allergic patient.

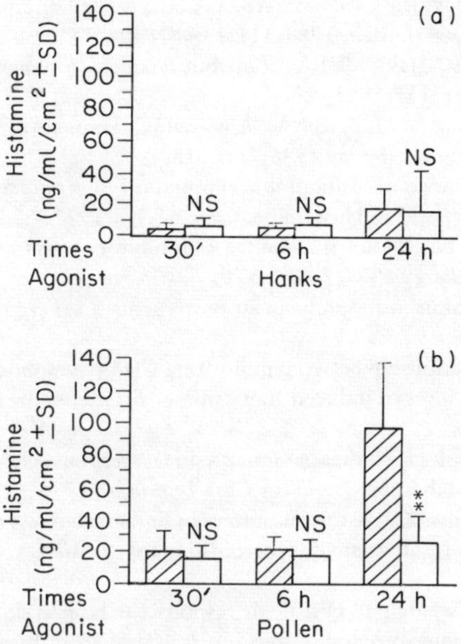

Fig. 13.7. Skin chamber technique in eight pollen-sensitive subjects. Measurement of histamine content in the skin chamber fluid during a specific allergic response. (a) Control situation: chambers were filled with Hank's medium (1 ml/chamber) all the time. (b) Allergic challenge: chambers were filled with pollen extract (0.01 IR/ml Hanks/chamber) from time 0 until time 6 h, and with Hank's medium from time 6 h until time 24 h. (▨) Placebo, (□) cetirizine 10 mg b.i.d. NS = $p > 0.1$, ** = $0.001 \leq p \leq 0.01$.

Skin studies offer a useful alternative to inhalation challenge when studying the phenomenon of cellular allergen-induced inflammation and the pharmacological modulation. Caution is naturally required when extrapolating results obtained on the skin to the use of the drug in asthma. Numerous investigations will be required to define the pharmacological properties profile of an ideal drug, in its action on different models of allergic reaction and inflammation.

Only controlled clinical trials can, however, help to evaluate the therapeutic benefits of the selected drug.

References

1 Fowler JW III, Lowell FC. The accumulation of eosinophils as an allergic response to allergen applied to the denuded skin surface. *J. Allergy Clin. Immunol.* 1966;37:19–28.

2 Rebuck JW, Crowley JH. A method of studying leukocytic functions *in vivo*. *Ann. NY Acad. Sci.* 1955;59:757–805.

3 Ting S, Dunsky EH, Lavker RM, Zweiman B. Patterns of mast cell alterations and *in vivo* mediator release in human allergic skin reactions. *J. Allergy Clin. Immunol.* 1980;66:417–423.

4 Issekutz AC. Quantitation of acute inflammation in the skin: recent methodological advances and their application to the study of inflammatory reactions. *Surv. Synth. Pathol. Res.* 1983;1:89–110.

5 Durham SR, Carroll M, Walsh GM, Kay AB. Leukocyte activation in allergen induced late phase asthmatic reactions. *N. Engl. J. Med.* 1984;**311**:1398–1402.

6 Wei Y, Heghinian K, Bell RL, Jakschik BA. Contribution of macrophages to immediate hypersensitivity reaction. *J. Immunol.* 1986;**137**:1993–2000.

7 Capron A, Dessaint JP, Capron M, Joseph M, Ameisen JC, Tonnel AB. From parasites to allergy: a second receptor for IgE. *Immunol. Today* 1986;**7**:15–18.

8 Bryant DH, Kay AB. Cutaneous eosinophil accumulation in atopic and non atopic individuals: the effect of an ECF-A tetrapeptide and histamine. *Clin. Allergy* 1977;**7**:211–217.

9 Fadel R, Herpin-Richard N, Rihoux JP, Henocq E. Inhibitory effect of cetirizine 2HCl on eosinophil migration *in vivo*. *Clin. Allergy* 1987;**7**:373–379.

10 Henocq E, Vargaftig BB. Skin eosinophilia in atopic patients. *J. Allergy Clin. Immunol.* 1988;**81**:691–695.

11 Frew AJ, Kay AB. The relationship between infiltrating CD4+ lymphocytes, activated eosinophils and the magnitude of the allergen-induced late phase cutaneous reaction in man. *J. Immunol.* 1988;**141**:4158–4164.

12 Slott RI, Zweiman B. Histologic studies in human skin test responses to ragweed and compound 48/80. II. Effects of corticosteroid therapy. *J. Allergy Clin. Immunol.* 1975;**55**:232–240.

13 Zweiman B, Slott RI, Atkins PC. Histologic studies of human skin test responses to ragweed and compounds 48/80. III. Effects of alternate day steroid therapy. *J. Allergy Clin. Immunol.* 1976;**58**:657–663.

14 Dunsky EH, Atkins PC, Zweiman B. Histologic responses in human skin test reactions to ragweed. IV. Effects of a single intravenous injection of steroids. *J. Allergy Clin. Immunol.* 1977;**59**:142–146.

15 Ting S, Zweiman B, Lavker RM. Cromolyn does not modulate human allergic skin reactions *in vivo*. *J. Allergy Clin. Immunol.* 1983;**71**:12–17.

16 Ting S, Zweiman B, Lavker RM. Terbutaline modulation of human allergic skin reactions. *J. Allergy Clin. Immunol.* 1983;**71**:437–441.

17 Eidinger D, Wilkinson R, Rose B. A study of cellular responses in immune reactions utilizing the skin window technique. *J. Allergy* 1964;**35**:77–85.

18 Michel L, De Vos C, Rihoux JP, Burtin C, Benveniste J, Dubertret L. Inhibitory effect of oral cetirizine on *in vivo* antigen induced histamine and PAF-acether release and eosinophil recruitment in human skin. *J. Allergy Clin. Immunol.* 1988;**82**:101–109.

19 Charlesworth EN, Kagey-Sobotka A, Norman PS, Lichtenstein LM. Effects of cetirizine on mast cell mediator release and cellular traffic during the cutaneous late phase response. *J. Allergy Clin. Immunol.* 1989;**83**:905–912.

20 Fadel R, Herpin-Richard N, Henocq E, Rihoux JP. Effect of cetirizine on *in vivo* cutaneous leukocyte migration in allergic rhinitis. *J. Allergy Clin. Immunol.* 1988;**81**:178.

21 De Vos C, Joseph M, Leprevost C, Vorng H, Tomassini M, Capron M, Capron A. Inhibition of human eosinophil chemotaxis and of the IgE dependent stimulation of human blood platelets by cetirizine. *Int. Arch. Allergy Appl. Immunol.* 1989;**88**:212–215.

22 Simons FE, Simons KJ, Chung M, Yeh J. The comparative pharmacokinetics of H1 receptor antagonists. *Ann. Allergy* 1987;**59**:20–24.

23 Leprevost C, Capron M, De Vos C, Tomassini M, Capron A. Inhibition of eosinophil chemotaxis by a new antiallergic compounds (cetirizine). *Int. Arch. Allergy Appl. Immunol.* 1988;**87**:9–13.

24 Roberts NM, Page CP, Chung KF, Barnes PJ. Effects of a PAF antagonist, BN 52063, on antigen-induced acute and late-onset cutaneous responses in atopic subjects. *J. Allergy Clin. Immunol.* 1988;**82**:236–241.

25 Kurihara K, Wardlaw AJ, Moqbel R, Kay AB. The ginkgolide (BN 52021) inhibits PAF induced chemotaxis and specific binding to human eosinophils and neutrophils. *J. Allergy Clin. Immunol.* 1988;**81**:208.

26 Ting S, Mansfield LE, Rauls DO. Failure of verapamil in inhibiting allergen induced histamine release *in vivo*. *Allergy* 1985;**40**:519–522.

27 Ting S, Rauls DO, Reiman BEF. Inhibitory effect of hydroxyzine on antigen induced histamine release *in vivo*. *J. Allergy Clin. Immunol.* 1985;75:63–66.

28 Atkins P, Shalit M, von Allmen C, Valenzano M, Zweiman B. *In vivo* and *in vitro* correlates of *in vivo* skin chamber histamine release. *J. Allergy Clin. Immunol.* 1988;**81**:297.

29 Shalit M, Schwartz LB, von Allmen C, Valenzano M, Atkins P, Kaliner M, Zweiman B. *In vivo* histamine and tryptase release during continuous and interrupted antigen challenge. *J. Allergy Clin. Immunol.* 1988;**81**:297.

30 Shalit M, Schwartz LB, Golzar N, von Allman C, Valenzano M, Fleekop P, Atkins PC, Zweiman B. Release of histamine and tryptase *in vivo* after prolonged cutaneous challenge with allergen in humans. *J. Immunol.* 1988;**141**:821–826.

31 Michel L, Jean-Louis F, De Vos C, Burtin C, Maclouf J, Dubertret L. Quantitative analysis of anaphylactic skin reactions *in vivo* in allergic patients. *Skin Pharmacol.* 1988;**1**:52.

14 · Platelet-activating factor and cutaneous eosinophilia

E. Hénocq* and B.B. Vargaftig

Introduction

Molecules produced during allergic inflammatory reactions attract eosinophils to the target organ and stimulate them to secrete [1]. Eosinophil products include platelet-activating factor (PAF)-acether [2,3], a mediator that duplicates different features of immediate hypersensitivity [4] including bronchoconstriction [5]. Conversely PAF may serve as a natural mediator for eosinophil participation in inflammatory and allergic reactions [6].

The skin cell content following a challenge with chemical or allergic stimulants can be evaluated by the skin window method of Rebuck and Crowley [7]. This *in vivo* test is available to the clinician who can follow the time-course of the skin reaction by its cellular effects. The test is performed by making a slight abrasion in the horny layer of the epidermis at the site of epicutaneous or intracutaneous application of the test product. A glass slide is then placed over the abraded area, attached with adhesive tape, and left in place for a variable period according to the established protocol. The slide is then stained (May–Grunwald–Giemsa), allowing the various cell populations of the inflammatory exudate, which have migrated to and settled on the underside of the slide, to be determined. Since it was first proposed by Rebuck [17], this test has been performed successfully by various authors in the domain of allergy [8–10]. Using this test, we showed that in response to PAF eosinophils accumulate in human skin of allergic patients only, whereas neutrophils were located in non-atopic controls.

Gross appearances of cutaneous reaction to PAF

An intradermal injection of 50 μl of a human serum albumin solution containing 200 ng of PAF (Bachem, Switzerland) elicits a biphasic inflammatory response similar to that induced by moderate doses of allergens in sensitized individuals [11]. In our preliminary studies, PAF and allergens elicited weal and flare responses that peaked within around 15 min. The diameters of the weal and flare induced by allergens in atopic patients were very similar to those induced by PAF. The acute inflammatory response was followed by a small area of erythema at the site of the resolved weal 24 h after the intradermal injection of PAF but no induration was observed. In non-

*Reprints from Dr E. Hénocq, 38 Rue Beaujon, 75008, Paris, France.

atopic controls the weal and flare reactions to PAF were very similar to those of atopic patients [12].

Microscopic studies

In contrast to the moderate macroscopic late-phase reaction, the atopic patients demonstrated a late (24 h) eosinophilic response to the allergens and to PAF. Many ruptured eosinophils were observed with free granules; in one-third up to almost half of the eosinophils were intensively degranulated. When assessing the eosinophil response, basophil leucocytes and free granules were noted in some, but not in all, preparations from atopic patients, but neither the presence nor the absence of basophils, or their number correlated with the number of eosinophils. In comparison very few, if any, eosinophils were observed in the non-atopic patients, where most cells present were neutrophils (60–70%) and mononuclear cells (macrophages and lymphocytes, 30–40%). In contrast, the cellular response in the control sites injected with the solvents alone showed only the usual inflammatory response induced by the skin window test itself, chiefly composed of neutrophils in non-atopic patients with very few eosinophils (about 1%) in atopic patients [12].

FMLP-induced skin eosinophilia

In atopic patients striking eosinophil responses were observed on skin sites challenged not only with allergens and PAF, but also with 5 μg of the peptide formyl-L-methionyl-L-leucyl-L-phenylalanine (FMLP). This soluble bacterial factor is chemotactic for neutrophils in normal controls [14]. The selective effect of FMLP on eosinophils from allergic controls agrees with the production of chemiluminescence by eosinophils from patients with moderate eosinophilia, in contrast to normal subjects when blood leucocytes are incubated with PAF or FMLP [15].

The phagocytosis of free eosinophilic granules by skin macrophages was also observed, as noted for lung tissue with respect to alveolar macrophages [13,16,17]. Eosinophils isolated from patients with hypereosinophilia release PAF in a dose and calcium-dependent manner when they are stimulated with eosinophil chemotactic factors of anaphylaxis, FMLP, or the calcium ionophore A23187, suggesting that chemotactic stimulation of eosinophils may be closely related to the biosynthesis and release of PAF [18].

Substance P-induced skin responses

In a preliminary study we observed weal and flare reactions in atopic as well as in non-atopic subjects upon the local application of the neuropeptide substance P, as reported previously [19,20]. It has been known since Lewis (1927) [21], that the introduction of histamine into human skin causes a triple reaction. The peripheral erythema can however be completely inhibited by prior application of capsaicin, a substance that depletes the skin of substance P [22]. On the other hand, intradermal injection of this neuropeptide produces papulo-erythematous reactions comparable with those provoked by histamine [19,20].

The erythema induced by intradermal injection of substance P (50 μl of a phosphate-buffered solution containing 50 pmol of substance P (Novobiochem, Switzerland) is inhibited by an antagonist of the histamine H_1 receptor. The papule, on the other hand, is either reduced or not modified [22]. Thus the neuropeptide released by the sensory nerve by axon reflex does not act directly to produce the vasodilation of the erythema, but rather indirectly, via histamine release by mast-cells [23]. In this case, histamine is the mediator of the erythema and not substance P itself [24].

We furthermore observed that the skin response to substance P includes an influx of activated macrophages, 24 h later, with numerous vacuoles, pseudopodes and figures of phagocytosis of granules. Polymorphonuclear neutrophils (PMN) are also noted and, in allergic patients, eosinophils as well. By contrast, in non-allergic subjects no eosinophils are seen. The significance of this influx of mononuclear cells and particularly of activated macrophages evoked preferentially by substance P has not been clearly established. The mechanism by which substance P induces the margination and the adhesion of PMN leucocytes and monocytes to the endothelium of venules remains obscure [25]. Nevertheless, it has been shown that the macrophage has on its surface receptor sites with a high affinity for substance P, which accounts for the release of pro-inflammatory and immunomodulating substances in response to substance P [26].

Macroscopic and microscopic skin responses to antisera specific for human IgE antibody

It is known from the work of the Ishizakas that only antibody/anti-IgE complexes can provoke immediate skin reactions in man when injected into the human skin [27]. We obtained with this reverse type allergic reaction (intradermal injection of 50 μl of a phosphate buffered solution containing goat anti-human IgE antibody (Fc) at 1/1000 dilution (Nordic Immunology, Tilburg, The Netherlands)) the same immediate hypersensitivity reactions in our allergic patients as described previously with the allergens, with PAF, FMLP and substance P. The macroscopic reactions often lasted as long as 6 h and after 24 h an influx of activated eosinophils compared with previous descriptions was noted. In contrast, in non-atopic subjects, despite the similar morphological appearance of the weal and flare reactions, the cellular response consisted mainly of PMN neutrophils and of monocytes/macrophages, but not of eosinophils. These observations correlate well with an *in vitro* activation of blood eosinophils from patients infected with filariae when incubated with specific antigen or anti-IgE antibody [28].

Discussion

Dual type reaction of intracutaneous PAF at 200 ng was characterized by a typical immediate weal and flare reaction followed by a late erythematous response of low intensity and free from induration or tenderness (at higher concentrations late cutaneous reactions to PAF are well documented [29]). Nevertheless, the skin eosinophilic response to PAF at 24 h was constantly observed irrespective of the presence or absence of a late allergic cutaneous reaction; this suggested that eosinophils are recruited into the lesions in concert with the development of a cellular late response in the majority of atopic patients [29].

Skin eosinophilotaxis was also observed in response to FMLP after 24 h. The marked chemotactic activity toward eosinophils in atopic subjects suggests a histamine-releasing capacity of FMLP-activated eosinophils by an IgE-independent mechanism [see also 31]. Aerosolization of FMLP induces dose-dependent bronchoconstriction in the guinea pig; this bronchoconstriction is accompanied by the activation, accumulation and aggregation of alveolar macrophages in the alveolar spaces and the presence of platelet micro-aggregates and of non-degranulated eosinophils [32]. Stimulated alveolar macrophages secrete inflammatory mediators including eosinophilotactic substances and thus participate in the pulmonary defence mechanisms [32]. A similar stimulation of macrophages has also been observed by us in human skin after an intradermal injection of substance P, PMN neutrophils being also observed and, in allergic patients only, eosinophils in moderate numbers. Thus cell activation occurs in tissue sites close to allergic and inflammatory lesions, and the majority of activated cells and their secretion products are on the sites of tissue damage [33]. Since macrophages can move from one body compartment to another and might thus serve as a kind of 'mobile synapse' conveying information from one body compartment to another through a physical translocation [34], the presence of a prominent influx of activated macrophages 24 h after an intracutaneous injection of substance P deserves attention, particularly since these cells have on their surface receptor sites with a high affinity for substance P [26].

The dose of allergen is a major factor in producing a late cutaneous allergic reaction (LCAR), which is a usual sequela of IgE-dependent reactions of sufficient intensity. The dose of allergens required for the development of a LCAR is in excess of the minimum requirement for a weal and flare reaction [35]. In our study, antibody/anti-IgE complexes, as well as the other chemoattractants previously described, were used at concentrations sufficient to induce appreciable weal and flare immediate reactions, but the LCAR were usually modest, in contrast to the eosinophilic responses which were of sufficient intensity, in response to the four products used in atopic subjects. By contrast, no eosinophils were seen in non-atopic controls, but only neutrophils and mononuclear cells, although the immediate type weal and flare reactions were of similar intensity in both groups. Cytophilic IgE is not restricted to cells with high affinity FcεRI receptors but is also detected with low affinity IgE receptors such as eosinophils [28]. IgE-bearing eosinophils can thus be activated to release pharmacological mediators by specific antigen or antisera specific for human IgE [36]. The anti-IgE-induced skin eosinophilia in atopic patients, as studied by the Rebuck skin window, offers the possibility of a new *in vivo* test available for the detection of atopy and related diseases with eosinophilia. Moreover, it is a useful tool to evaluate the effects of drugs on the skin and to correlate with their underlying cellular components in comparative studies with other chemoattractants.

References

1 Spry CJF. *Eosinophils.* Oxford University Press, 1988.

2 Lee T, Lenihan DJ, Malone B, Roddy LL, Wasserman SI. Increased biosynthesis of platelet-activating factor in activated human eosinophils. *J. Biol. Chem.* 1984;**259**:5526.

3 Jouvin-Marche E, Grzych JM, Boullet C, Capron M, Benveniste J. Formation of paf-acether by human eosinophils (abstract). *Fed. Proc.* 1984;**43**:1924.

4 Braquet P, Touqui L, Shen, Vargaftig BB. Perspectives in platelet-activating factor research. *Pharmacol. Rev.* 1987;**39**:97.

5 Vargaftig BB, Lefort J, Chignard M, Benveniste J. Platelet-activating factor induces a platelet-dependent bronchoconstriction unrelated to the formation of prostaglandin derivatives. *Eur. J. Pharmacol.* 1980; **65**:185.

6 Morley J, Page CP, Sanjar S. The platelet in asthma. *Lancet* 1984;ii:1142–1144.

7 Rebuck JW, Crowley JH. A method of studying leukocytic functions *in vivo*. *Ann. NY Acad. Sci.* 1955;**54**:757.

8 Eidinger D, Wilkinson R, Rose B. A study of cellular responses in immune reactions utilizing the skin window technique. I. Immediate hypersensitivity reactions. *J. Allergy Clin. Immunol.* 1971;**48**:125–133.

9 Fowler JW III, Lowel FC. The accumulation of eosinophils as an allergic response to allergen applied to the denuded skin surface. *J. Allergy Clin. Immunol.* 1966;**37**:19.

10 Felarca AB, Lowel FC. The accumulation of eosinophils and basophils in skin sites as related to intensity of skin reactivity and symptoms in atopic disease. *J. Allergy Clin. Immunol.* 1971;**48**(3):125–133.

11 Wardlaw AJ, Moqbel R, Cromwell O, Kay AB. Platelet-activating factor: a potent chemotactic and chemokinetic factor for human eosinophils. *J. Clin. Invest.* 1986;**78**:1701–1706.

12 Hénocq E, Vargaftig BB. Accumulation of eosinophils in response to intracutaneous PAF-acether and allergen in man. *Lancet* 1986;i:1379.

13 Hénocq E, Vargaftig BB. Skin eosinophilia in atopic patients. *J. Allergy Clin. Immunol.* 1988;**81**(4):691–695.

14 Marasco WA, Phan SH, Krutzsch H, Showell HJ, Feltner EL, Nalm R, Becker ZL, Ward PA. Purification and identification of formyl-methionyl-leucyphenylalanine as the major peptide neutrophil chemotactic factor produced by *Escherichia coli*. *J. Biol. Chem.* 1984;**259**:5430.

15 Bruijnzeel PLB, Koenderman L, Verhaegen J. Chemoluminescence by eosinophils from normals and patients with moderate eosinophilia (abstract). *Ann. Allergy* 1985;**55**:250.

16 Lellouch-Tubiana A, Lefort J, Simon MT, Pfister A, Vargaftig BB. Eosinophil recruitment into guinea-pig lungs after PAF-acether and allergen administration: modulation of prostacyclin, platelet depletion, and selective antagonists. *Am. Rev. Respir. Dis.* 1988;**137**:948–954.

17 Tonnel AB, Prin M, Capron M, Wallaert B, Capron A. Infiltrats pulmonaires d'éosinophiles: étude comparée des éosinophiles sanguins et alvéolaires In: *Traitement de l'asthme* (Eds Godard P, Bousquet J, Michel FB) Masson Publishing, Paris: 1985.

18 Ten-Ching L, Lenihan DJ, Malone B, Roddy LL, Wasserman SI. Increased biosynthesis of platelet-activating-factor in activated human eosinophils. *J. Biol. Chem.* 1984;**259**:5526–5530.

19 Hägermark Ö, Hökfelt T, Pernow B. Flare and itch induced by substance P in human skin. *J. Invest. Dermatol.* 1978;**71**:233–235.

20 Fewtrell CMS, Foreman JC, Jordan CC, Oehme P, Renner H, Stewart JM. The effect of substance P on histamine and 5-hydroxytryptamine release in human skin. *J. Physiol.* 1982;**330**:313–411.

21 Lewis T. *The Blood Vessels of the Human Skin and their Responses.* Shaw and sons, London, 1927.

22 Foreman JC, Jordan CC, Oehmer P, Renner H. Structure activity relationships for some substance P-related peptides that cause wheal and flare reactions in human skin. *J. Physiol.* 1983;**335**:449–465.

23 Barnes PJ, Brown MJ, Dollery CT, Fuller RW, Heavey DJ, Ind PW. Histamine is released from skin by substance P but does not act as the final vasodilator in the axon reflex. *Br. J. Pharmac.* 1986;**88**:741–745.

24 Foreman JF. Neuropeptides and the pathogenesis of allergy. *Allergy* 1987;**212**:1–11.

25 Goetzl EJ, Chernov T, Renold KV. Neuropeptide regulation of the expression of immediate hypersensitivity. *J. Immunol.* 1985;**135**(2):802S–805S.

26 Hartung HP, Wolters K, Toyka KV. Substance P: binding properties and studies on cellular responses in guinea pig macrophages. *J. Immunol.* 1986;**136**(10):3856–3863.

27 Ishizaka K, Ishizaka T. Skin reactions by anti-E globulin antibodies in humans and monkeys. *J. Immunol.* 1968;**100**(3):554–562.

28 Capron M, Kusniecz JP, Prin L, Spiegelberg HL, Khalife J, Tonnel AB, Capron A. Cytophilic IgE on human blood and tissue eosinophils. *Int. Arch. Allergy Appl. Immun.* 1985;**77**:246–248.

29 Archer CB, Page CP, Morley J, Macdonald DM. Accumulation of inflammatory cells in response to intracutaneous platelet activating factor (Paf-acether) in man. *Br.J. Dermatol.* 1985;**112**:285–290.

30 Sollers GO, Gleich GJ, Jordan RE, Schroeter AL. Late phase of the immediate weal and flare skin reaction: its dependence on IgE antibodies. *J. Clin. Invest.* 1976;**58**:408.

31 Conroy MC, Kennedy JA, Thueson DO. Differential inhibition of histamine release from human basophils induced by antigen, anti-IgE, or *N*-formy-L-methionyl-L-leucyl-L-phenylalanine. *Int. Arch. Allergy Appl. Immunol.* 1985;**77**:222.

32 Boukili MA, Bureau MF, Lellouch-Tubiana A, Lefort J, Simon MT, Vargaftig BB. Alveolar macrophages and eicosanoids but not neutrophils mediate bronchoconstriction induced by FMLP in the guinea-pig. *Br. J. Pharmacol.* 1989;**98**:61.

33 Spry CF, Tai PC, Barkans J. Tissue localization of human eosinophil cationic proteins in allergic diseases. *Int. Arch. Allergy Appl. Immunol.* 1985;**77**:252–254.

34 Norcross MA. A synaptic basis for T-lymphocytes-activation. *Ann. Immunol. (Paris)* 1984;**135D**:112.

35 Limenoto L, Poothullil J, Dolovich J, Hargreave FE. Factors which influence late cutaneous allergic responses. *J. Allergy Clin. Immunol.* 1976;**58**:60–68.

36 Moqbel R, Walsh GM, Macdonald AJ, Kay B. Effect of disodium cromoglycate on activation of human eosinophils and neutrophils following reversed (anti-IgE) anaphylaxis. *Clin. Allergy* 1986;**16**:73–83.

15 · Eosinophils, T-lymphocytes and late-phase skin reactions

A.J. Frew

Introduction

Since the end of the 19th century it has been recognized that sensitive subjects can develop acute symptoms of asthma and/or rhinitis when exposed to inhalant allergens [1]. In many atopic subjects there follows a delayed and more prolonged reaction, the late-phase allergic reaction (LPR). Such LPRs may be seen in the lungs, nose, skin and conjunctiva. Clinical scientists have been interested in the LPR for several reasons: firstly, LPRs are associated with more severe clinical symptoms; secondly, the physiology and pharmacology of the late-phase response are close to those of 'real life asthma,' which is not true of the immediate response to allergen. This implies that at least some of the events occurring in the LPR model are relevant to the disease process. Most importantly, experimental LPRs to allergen make it possible to study the chemical and cellular events of allergic inflammation in a controlled and reproducible fashion [2].

Though the bronchoconstriction of the late asthmatic reaction is at least partially due to smooth-muscle contraction, it is clear that other events are also relevant as simple bronchodilators are less effective in the late-phase compared with the early phase. In animal models, late asthmatic reactions are characterized histologically by a combination of bronchial mucosal oedema and cellular infiltration. Such histological studies have not been performed in man, but human bronchoalveolar lavage (BAL) studies reveal accumulation of eosinophils, mononuclear cells and neutrophils [3,4].

It is clearly of great interest and importance to consider how these cells are recruited and how their actions may be regulated. The initial response following allergen challenge seems to be mediated through the release of chemical mediators from cells bearing Fc receptors for IgE. Mast-cell mediators can certainly induce local and non-specific changes in vascular permeability; this may account for the initial localization of cells at allergic reaction sites and the first stages of their migration into the tissue. Chemotactic factors released by mast-cells have been extensively studied, but these seem to be more active towards neutrophils except for PAF which is active on both neutrophils and eosinophils *in vitro* [5]. Mast-cell mediator release cannot therefore account for the specificity of the changes observed. In addition, there is only a modest correlation between the size of the early and late-phase reactions in the human skin [6,7] while it is impossible to predict the magnitude of the late asthmatic response from the size of the early asthmatic response [8].

Recent evidence from *in vitro* studies has indicated that T-lymphocyte-derived mediators can selectively attract and stimulate eosinophils [9,10] and can prolong eosinophil survival in culture, especially in the presence of fibroblasts [11–13]. From this work there is now an emerging consensus that T-lymphocyte products may be an important element in the regulation of allergic inflammation, as well as controlling the IgE antibody production [14].

Cellular accumulation in the human cutaneous LPR

We have conducted a study of the cellular events of the human late-phase allergic reaction in order to determine the nature of the cellular infiltrate and to examine whether T-cell accumulation might account for the specificity of the cellular changes [15].

Cutaneous late-phase skin reactions (CLPR) were induced in a group of subjects with atopic rhinitis, by intradermal challenge with 30 BU *Dermatophagoides pteronyssinus* or grass pollen extract. The diameter of the CLPR was measured at 6 h and skin biopsies were obtained after 6, 24 or 48 h (10 subjects at each timepoint) using lignocaine anaesthesia. The phenotypes of infiltrating leucocytes were determined by immunocytochemistry and a panel of monoclonal antibodies.

Neutrophils were seen in considerable numbers at 6 h but there was no correlation between the degree of neutrophil infiltration and CLPR size ($r = 0.02$). By 24 h, neutrophils had largely disappeared. Substantial numbers of eosinophils were detected in the allergen challenged sites by staining with the acidic dye Chromotrope 2R. To assess eosinophil activation, the monoclonal antibody EG2 was employed. This antibody recognizes an epitope which is present on the secreted forms of eosinophil cationic protein and eosinophil derived neurotoxin [16] and which is not expressed on resting blood eosinophils. Activated eosinophils, stained with EG2, were present in the allergen challenged sites at all three timepoints and comparing the number of cells stained with Chromotrope and EG2, it was apparent that the vast majority of eosinophils in the dermis were activated.

At 6 h there was no association between the number of activated eosinophils and the magnitude of the CLPR. However, an association emerged during the experiments between the magnitude of the CLPR measured at 6 h and the persistence of activated eosinophils. This implies that there are either common or proportional mechanisms involved in the expression of the CLPR and in the persistence of activated eosinophils in tissue. Monocyte accumulation was assessed by staining for non-specific esterase and with a CD14 monoclonal antibody. Both methods revealed a small elevation in monocyte numbers at allergen challenged sites, but this was not statistically significant compared with the saline challenged control sites.

Whereas eosinophils and neutrophils were seen scattered through the dermis, T-lymphocyte accumulation was more localized, in and around the dermal small blood vessels. T-lymphocyte numbers were significantly increased at all three timepoints, with a slight decrease over 48 h. Subset analysis revealed the majority of these T-lymphocytes to be CD4+ (i.e. helper/inducer T-cells). Some T-cells expressed interleukin-2 (IL-2) receptors (CD25 or Tac) indicating activation. Interleukin-2R+ cells constituted between 0 and 15% of the total T-lymphocyte numbers and there were statistically significant differences from control sites at 24 and 48 h but not at 6 h. Additional, indirect evidence of local T-cell activation was furnished by the presence of HLA-DR staining on endothelial cells and CD4 staining on Langerhans cells after 24 and 48 h, both these phenomena being consistent with the local secretion of interferon (IFN)γ [17,18].

Small numbers of CD8+ cells were detected but with no statistical difference from control sites. Furthermore, there was no association between the CD4/CD8 ratios in the peripheral blood and in the tissue, confirming that the infiltrate was indeed selective for CD4+ cells.

There was no direct correlation between CLPR size and T-cell numbers at any of the timepoints studied, but interestingly there was a striking association between the number of CD4+ T-cells and the number of activated eosinophils at 24 h ($r = 0.94$, $p < 0.001$) suggesting that T-lymphocytes may be regulating the persistence of activated eosinophils in the tissue.

Discussion

There is a wealth of *in vitro* evidence suggesting that eosinophil granule products contribute to the pathogenesis of allergic inflammation [19]. Monocyte products may also cause local damage to the bronchial epithelium. It is also conceivable that T-cells may have direct effects on epithelial cells through as yet undefined mechanisms. On the other hand T-cells generally act as regulators and amplifiers of the immune response and it is reasonable to conclude that T-cells are involved in regulating the allergic response.

T-cells clearly play an important part in allergic inflammation by their regulation of IgE production, via the lymphokines IL-4 and IFN-γ [14]. It is now apparent that T-cell products can enhance the survival of eosinophils in culture, and by implication *in vivo* [11,12]. Furthermore, lymphokines can locally upregulate the function of eosinophils, neutrophils and mononuclear phagocytes [20].

Finally, it is important to remember that the primary purpose of any inflammatory process is to deal with a perceived external threat to the organism. It seems likely that the allergic inflammatory response does not exist in order to produce disease, but is rather a complex defence mechanism whose ideal outcome is resolution rather than persistent inflammation. As such the allergic response presumably stimulates repair processes which may involve fibroblasts and counterinflammatory cells: our present knowledge of these areas is rudimentary and there is clearly much work to do.

References

1 Blackley C. *Experimental Researches on the Causes and Nature of Catarrhus Aestivus (Hayfever or Asthma)*. Baillieré Tindall & Cox 1873, pp. 77–81; reprinted by Dawsons of Pall Mall, London 1959.

2 Gleich GJ. The late phase of the immunoglobulin E-mediated reaction: a link between anaphylaxis and common allergic disease. *J. Allergy Clin. Immunol.* 1982;**70**:160–169.

3 De Monchy JGR, Kauffman HF, Venge P, Koeter GH, Jansen HM, Sluiter HR, de Vries K. Bronchoalveolar eosinophilia during allergen induced late asthmatic reactions. *Am. Rev. Respir. Dis.* 1985;**131**:373–376.

4 Metzger WJ, Zavala D, Richerson HB, Moseley P, Iwamota P, Monick M. Sjoerdsma K, Hunninghake GW. Local allergen challenge and bronchoalveolar lavage of allergic asthmatic lungs. Description of the model and local airway inflammation. *Am. Rev. Respir. Dis.* 1987;**135**:433–440.

5 Wardlaw AJ, Moqbel R, Cromwell O, Kay AB. Platelet activating factor. A potent chemotactic and chemokinetic factor for human eosinophils. *J. Clin. Invest.* 1986;**78**:1701–1706.

6 Rocklin RE. Clinical and immunologic aspects of allergen specific immunotherapy in patients with seasonal allergic rhinitis and/or allergic asthma. *J. Allergy Clin. Immunol.* 1983;**72**:323–334.

7 Frew AJ, Kay AB. The pattern of human late phase skin reactions to extracts of aeroallergens. *J. Allergy Clin. Immunol.* 1988a;**81**:1117–1121.

8 Cartier A, Thomson NC, Frith PA, Roberts R, Hargreave FE. Allergen induced increase in bronchial responsiveness to histamine: relationship to the late asthmatic response and change in airway caliber. *J. Allergy Clin. Immunol.* 1982; **70**:171–177.

9 Lopez AF, Sanderson CJ, Gamble JR, Campbell HD, Young IG, Vadas MA. Recombinant human interleukin-5 is a selective activator of human eosinophil function. *J. Exp. Med.* 1988;**167**:219–224.

10 Yamaguchi Y, Hayashi Y, Sugama Y, Miura Y, Kasaharu T, Kitamura S, Torisu M, Mita S, Tominaga A, Takatsu K, Suda T. Highly purified murine IL-5 stimulates eosinophil function and prolong *in vitro* survival. IL-5 as a chemotactic factor. *J. Exp. Med.* 1988;**167**:1737–1742.

11 Owen WF, Rothenburg ME, Silberstein DS, Gasson JC, Stevens RL, Austen KF, Soberman RJ. Regulation of human eosinophil viability, density and function by granulocyte/macrophage colony stimulating factor in the presence of 3T3 fibroblasts. *J. Exp. Med.* 1987;**166**:129–141.

12 Rothenburg ME, Owen WF, Silberstein DS, Soberman RJ, Austen KF, Stevens RL. Eosinophils co-cultured with endothelial cells have increased survival and functional properties. *Science* 1987;**237**:645–647.

13 Saito H, Hatake K, Dvorak AM, Leiferman KM, Donnenberg AD, Arai N, Ishizaka K, Ishizaka T. Selective induction of differentiation and proliferation of haematopoietic cells by recombinant human interleukins. *Proc. Natl. Acad. Sci. USA* 1988;**85**:2288–2292.

14 Teale JM, Abraham KM. The regulation of antibody class expression. *Immunol. Today* 1987;**8**:122.

15 Frew AJ, Kay AB. The relationship between activated eosinophils, CD4+ T lymphocytes and allergen-induced late phase skin reactions in man. *J. Immunol.* 1988b;**141**:4158–4164.

16 Tai P–C, Spry CJF, Peterson C, Verge P, Olsson I.Monoclonal antibodies distinguish between storage and secreted forms of eosinophil cationic protein. *Nature* **309**:182–184.

17 Walsh LJ, Parry A, Scholes A, Seymour GJ. Modulation of CD4 antigen on human gingival langerhans cells by gamma interferon. *Clin. Exp. Immunol.* 1987;**70**:379–382.

18 Hirschberg H, Braathen LR, Thorsby E. Antigen presentation by vascular endothelical cells and epidermal langerhans cells: the role of HLA-DR. *Immunol. Rev.* 1982;**66**:57–77.

19 Wardlaw AJ, Kay AB. The role of the eosinophil in the pathogenesis of asthma. *Allergy* 1987;**42**:321–335.

20 Miyajima A, Miyatake S, Schreurs J, de Vries J, Arai N. Yokota T, Arai K. Coordinate regulation of immune and inflammatory responses by T cell derived lymphokines. *FASEB J.* 1988;**2**:2462–2473.

16 · Inhibition of PAF-induced eosinophilia by AH 21–132, a novel anti-asthma drug

J. Morley and I.D. Chapman

After guinea pigs have been exposed to an aerosol of platelet-activating factor (PAF), it is possible to demonstrate increased sensitivity of the airways to spasmogens, whether administered intravenously [1], or by inhalation [2]. In addition, it can be shown that there is a selective infiltration of eosinophils into the lumen of intrapulmonary airways of these animals [3].

Development of airway hyperreactivity following exposure to PAF may be dissociated from pulmonary eosinophilia, since bronchial hyperreactivity due to PAF is absolutely dependent on platelet activation, becomes apparent within 10 min, and ceases to be evident by about 24 h [1]; eosinophil accumulation, on the other hand, is of slower onset, not maximal until 48 h have elapsed and not influenced by platelet depletion [3]. Thus, although eosinophil accumulation is associated with the development of increased reactivity of the airways, it cannot be presumed that epithelial damage by eosinophils has produced airway hyperreactivity; especially since at the time of maximal eosinophil infiltration, when there is clear evidence of epithelial desquamation, airway responsivity lies within the normal range. Such dichotomy is also a feature of the response to inhaled allergen in the guinea pig, for eosinophil accumulation can be demonstrated with or without airway hyperreactivity by varying the intensity of the allergic reaction [4]. Even though eosinophil activation may not be a primary determinant of airway hyperreactivity, it can be expected that impaired clearance of mucus and cellular debris will contribute to asthma pathology by causing inefficient ventilation of small airways, with impaired gas exchange and gas trapping. Consequently, it is of interest to ascertain whether anti-asthma drugs influence intrapulmonary eosinophil accumulation. As yet, few animal studies have been reported, even though there is clinical evidence that certain anti-asthma drugs are able to diminish eosinophilia in peripheral blood or sputum [5–7].

The mechanism whereby inhalation of allergen of PAF induces intrapulmonary eosinophilia in conscious guinea pigs has yet to be defined. Guinea pigs, like rats, breathe via the nose with the consequence that almost all inhaled material can be expected to be swallowed following deposition within extrapulmonary airways unless absorbed across the nasal epithelium [8]. The pulmonary eosinophilia that follows exposure to an aerosol of PAF may thus be a result of systemic absorption and the capacity of PAF to induce comparable intrapulmonary eosinophilia when injected into the peritoneal cavity [9] accords with this interpretation. Chemotaxis cannot account for this effect of PAF, since PAF is metabolized to lyso-PAF within a few minutes [10]. It must be concluded that exposure to PAF provides a brief but adequate signal for eosinophil mobilization, so that these cells effect tissue-specific mobilization by responding to chemotactic or other stimuli when within the lung vasculature.

Accumulation of eosinophils within the lungs of guinea pigs may be measured conveniently by airway lavage. Guinea pigs have been exposed for 1 h to an aerosol of PAF (10 μg/ml in saline containing 0.25% BSA), generated by a jet nebulizer using compressed air. Animals were killed with barbiturate after 48 h. Following tracheal cannulation, successive 10-ml aliquots of buffered modified Tyrode solution (composition mM: $NaHCO_3$ 11.9, NaCl 136.9, KCl 2.7, Na_2HPO_4 0.4, glucose 5.6, EDTA 19.8; protein % w/v: Gelatin 0.1, BSA 0.5; pH 7.4) were introduced successively and aspirated by gentle compression of the lung tissue; total fluid recovery normally exceeded 50 ml (80%). Cell suspensions were concentrated by low speed centrifugation (200 *g* for 10 min) and the resulting cell pellet was resuspended in 1 ml of modified Tyrode solution. Total cell counts were made by diluting 10 μl of cell suspension in 90 μl of Turks fluid. Differential cell counts were made from smears fixed in methanol (100%) and stained with Leishman stain. At least 500 cells/smear were counted at 1000-fold magnification, in order to differentiate cell types.

In order to ascertain the efficacy of anti-asthma drugs as inhibitors of pulmonary eosinophilia, drugs have been administered for 7 days as a sustained subcutaneous infusion from an implanted minipump (Alzet 2001 and 2ML1), so that exposure of PAF occurred only after a 5-day pretreatment period with the test compound. Administration of cromoglycate (1–10 mg/kg/day), ketotifen (0.1–10 mg/kg/day), theophylline (10 mg/kg/day) and dexamethasone (1–10 mg/kg/day) over 5 days prior to inhalation of PAF and 2 days thereafter, effected significant inhibition of pulmonary eosinophilia; conversely mepyramine (2 mg/kg/day), indomethacin (1 mg/kg/day) and salbutamol (1 mg/kg/day) proved ineffective. These results imply that airway eosinophilia as a reaction to PAF may constitute a test system appropriate for anti-asthma drug detection.

The benzonapthyridine, AH 21–132 (Fig. 16.1) is a mixture of two isomers, with biological activity being largely associated with the (−) isomer. Although structurally distinct from known anti-asthma drugs, AH 21–132 shares with ketotifen, dexamethasone, cromoglycate and theophylline, the capacity to inhibit development of airway hyperreactivity due to intravenous injection of PAF [11]. In order to ascertain whether this inhibitory activity extended to eosinophilia, AH 21–132 was administered from a subcutaneous osmotic minipump for 5 days prior to inhalation of PAF and 2 days thereafter. Doses of AH 21–132 between 0.1 and 1.0 mg/kg/day effected inhibition of eosinophil accumulation, hence the potency of AH 21–132 in this test system was comparable with ketotifen or dexamethasone when administered by this route (Table 16.1). Prolonged infusion of AH 21–132 (1 mg/kg/day) also inhibited eosinophil accumulation within the airway lumen of guinea pigs, which had been ac-

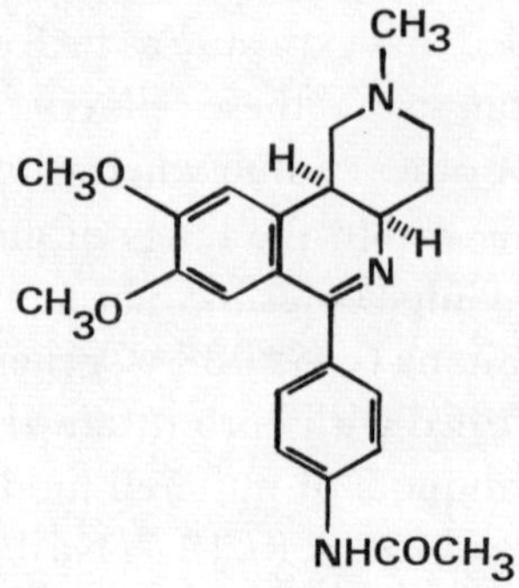

Fig. 16.1. AH 21–132. *cis*-6-(*p*-acetamidophenyl)-1,2,3,4,4*a*,10*b*-hexahydro-8,9-dimethoxy-2-methylbenzo[*c*] [1,6]-naphthyridine.

tively sensitized to ovalbumin and subjected to inhalation of allergen as an aerosol. Furthermore, in animals exhibiting idiopathic airway eosinophilia, repeated oral administration of AH 21–132 (1 mg/kg/day), like ketotifen (1 mg/kg/day), caused significant diminution of pulmonary eosinophilia (Table 16.1).

Table 16.1. The effect of AH 21–132, ketotifen and dexamethasone upon diverse forms of eosinophilia (n = 10)

Stimulus of eosinophilia	Drug dose (mg/kg/day)	AH 21–132	Ketotifen (% inhibition)	Dexamethasone
PAF	0.1	44	44	—
	1	57	57	60
Antigen	1	54	54	54
Idiopathic	1	53	53	63

The mechanism whereby AH 21–132 achieves inhibition of these diverse forms of eosinophilia remains to be defined. It is noteworthy that inhibitory effects are not restricted to PAF, but extend to other agencies including lymphokines and cytokines. In the guinea pig, intraperitoneal injection of recombinant lymphokines or cytokines can induce selective eosinophil accumulation comparable with that achieved by PAF; AH 21–132 proved able to inhibit these responses to a comparable degree. All of these effects of AH 21–132 cannot be attributed to antagonism of PAF since AH 21–132 fails to interact as a competitive antagonist at PAF binding sites; moreover selective antagonism of PAF is an improbable mechanism for inhibition of all forms of eosinophilia since PAF receptor antagonists do not inhibit allergen-induced airway eosinophilia in the guinea pig [9] nor do such compounds influence idiopathic eosinophilia. The ability of AH 21–132 to diminish eosinophilia irrespective of the activation stimulus is more readily explained by an action at the level of a second messenger system rather than as a receptor antagonist.

When it was observed that AH 21–132 could abrogate the development of airway hyperreactivity due to PAF, it became necessary to exclude bronchodilator activity as a basis for such biological activity. AH 21–132 had previously been subjected to a pharmacological analysis as a potential ionotropic drug, hence it was a surprising finding that AH 21–132 relaxed airway smooth-muscle, and also exerted a selective effect on this tissue. The bronchodilator effect of AH 21–132 cannot *per se* explain the capacity of AH 21–132 to inhibit development of airway hyperreactivity, since inhibitory effects considerably outlast the duration of bronchodilator efficacy. Definition of a biological activity that could be detected *in vitro* [12] was of considerable interest, since this finding allowed detailed analysis of one pharmacological effect of AH 21–132, with the possibility that there may be a common mechanism underlying airway smooth-muscle relaxation and altered eosinophil function.

The spasmolytic activity of AH 21–132 is unrelated to beta adrenoceptor agonist or parasympatholytic activity and cannot be attributed to selective antagonism of spasmogens of airway smooth muscle [12]; nor is it related to an effect upon transmembrane calcium or potassium channel activation [13]. It has been known for some time that AH 21–132, like theophylline, is a potent phosphodiesterase (PDE) inhibitor [14]; however, the action of AH 21–132 upon airway smooth-muscle can be distinguished from that of theophylline by the following criteria: AH 21–132 effected an enhanced relaxant action on airway smooth-muscle following epithelial removal whereas theophylline has no such effect [12]; AH 21–132 was without effect on isolated tracheal smooth-muscle maintained at 12°C, whereas theophylline induced spasm attributable to the release of calcium from intracellular stores [13]; AH 21–132, in contrast to theophylline, exhibited selectivity as an inhibitor of cAMP PDE as opposed to cGMP PDE derived from tracheal smooth-muscle [13]. On the other hand, inhibition of platelet cAMP PDE activity has not facilitated selection of structural analogues with spasmolytic efficacy comparable with AH 21–132 (Fig. 16.2). However, more recent evidence [15,16] has implicated inhibition of an isoenzyme, the type III PDE isolated from bovine trachea, as a site of action for AH 21–132. This enzyme comprises a minor proportion (~ 5%) of cAMP PDE of airway smooth-muscle yet may exert a decisive influence in the contractile response [17]. If the PDE isoenzyme of eosinophils or airway smooth-muscle is selectively inhibited by AH 21–132 then such an effect would be favoured to explain both relaxation of airway smooth-muscle and inhibition of eosinophilia.

Established prophylactic anti-asthma drugs such as ketotifen, cromoglycate and glucocorticosteroids lack bronchodilator activity. The inability of these drugs to provide immediate symptomatic relief may be considered a deficiency, since it is

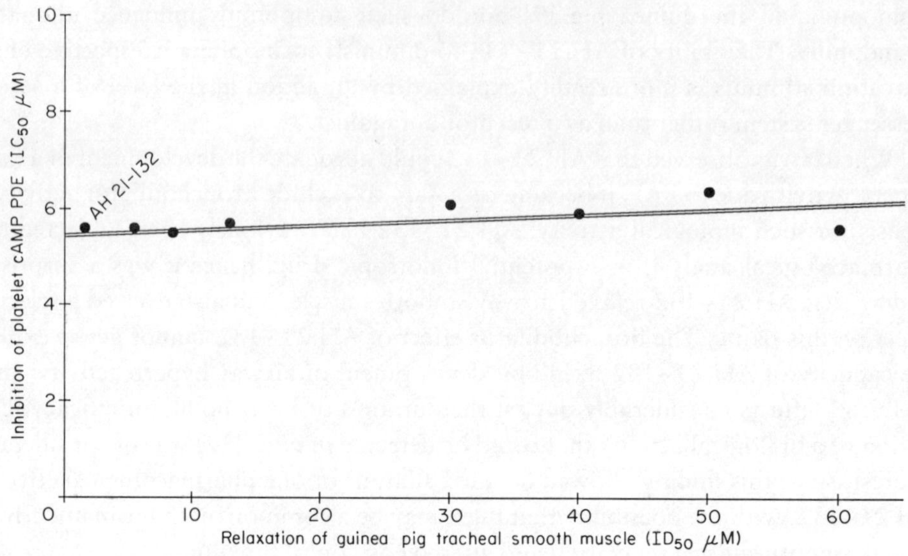

Fig. 16.2. Lack of correlation between inhibition of platelet cAMP PDE and airway smooth-muscle relaxation *in vitro* by analogues of AH 21–132.

apparent that disinclination to use prophylactic anti-asthma drugs may be related to an absence of perceived symptomatic benefit [18]. For this reason the combination of bronchodilator activity with impaired eosinophil accumulation is an attractive profile for an anti-asthma drug. An understanding of the biochemical events that account for this combination of properties in AH 21–132 will be of considerable importance; should AH 21–132 exert corresponding clinical benefits in asthma, there is a realistic prospect for rational selection of prophylactic anti-asthma drugs that have symptomatic benefit.

References

1 Mazzoni L, Morley J, Page CP, Sanjar S. Induction of airway hyperreactivity by platelet activating factor in the guinea-pig. *Br. J. Physiol.* 1985;**365**:107.

2 Fitzgerald MF, Leesi W, Parente L, Payne AN. Exposure to PAF-acether aerosol induces airway hyper-responsiveness in guinea-pigs. *Br. J. Pharm.* 1987;**90**:112.

3 Aoki S, Boubeker K, Burrows L, Morley J, Sanjar S. Recruitment of eosinophils by platelet activating factor (PAF) in the guinea-pig lung. *J. Physiol.* 1987;**394**:130.

4 Aoki S, Boubeker K, Kristersson A, Morley J, Sanjar S. Is allergic hyperreactivity of the guinea-pig dependent on eosinophil accumulation. *Br. J. Pharm.* 1988;**94**:365.

5 Horn BR, Robin ED, Theodore J, van Kessel A. Total eosinophil counts in the management of bronchial asthma. *New Engl. J. Med.* 1975;**292**:1152–1155.

6 Medici TC, Radielovic P, Steiner A. Short term effects of ketotifen in bronchial asthma. *Am. Rev. Resp. Dis.* 1980;**121**:85.

7 Diaz P, Galleguillos FR, Gonzalez MC, Pantin CFA, Kay AB. Bronchoalveolar lavage in asthma: the effect of disodium cromoglycate (cromolyn) on leucocyte counts, immunoglobulins and complement. *J. Allergy Clin. Immunol.* 1984;74:41–48.

8 Gazeley MJS, Lees IW, Payne AN, Webbon PM, Wooley GE. Anatomical deposition and early distribution of inhaled radioaerosol in conscious and anaesthetised rats. *Br. J. Pharm.* 1986;87:122.

9 Boubeker K, Morley J. Use of PAF antagonists to assess the role of PAF in allergen induced responses of the guinea-pig airway. *Prostaglandins* 1988;35:799.

10 Latrigue-Mattei C, Godeneche D, Chabard JL, Petie J, Berger JA. Pharmakokinetic study of ^{3}H labelled PAF-acether. II. Comparison with ^{3}H labelled lyso-PAF acether after intravenous administration in the rabbit and protein binding. *Agents Actions* 1984;15:643–648.

11 Kristersson A, Morley J, Schaeublin E. Properties of AH 21–132 that could contribute to prophylactic activity in asthma *Br. J. Pharm.* 1988;93:53.

12 Bewley JS, Chapman ID. AH 21–132: a novel relaxant of airway smooth muscle. *Br. J. Pharm.* 1988;93:52.

13 Boyle JP, Duty S, Elliot KRF, Foster RW, Small RC, Watt AJ. Mechanical, electrical and biochemical effects of AH 21–132 in guinea-pig isolated trachealis. *Br. J. Pharm.* 1989;96:161.

14 Markstein R, Digges K, Marshall NR, Starke K. Forskolin and the release of noradrenaline in cerebrocortical slices. *Naunyn Schmiedebergs Arch. Pharmacol.* 1984;325:17–24.

15 Berry JL, Boyle JP, Elliot KRF, Foster RW, Small RC, Watt AJ. Some mechanical and biochemical effects of AH 21–132 in guinea-pig cardiac tissue and bovine trachealis. *Br. J. Pharm.* 1989;97:446.

16 Glembycz MA, Mak JC, Ukena D, Chilvers ER, Barnes PJ. AH 21–132 inhibits type III/IV cyclic nucleotide dependent phosphodiesterase activity in bovine trachealis. *Br. J. Pharm.* 1989;97:559.

17 Torphy TJ. Action of mediators on airway smooth muscle: functional antagonism as a mechanism for bronchodilator drugs. In: Directions for new anti-asthma drugs. *Agents Actions* 1988; Suppl. 23:37–53.

18 Reed CE. New therapeutic approaches in asthma. *J. Allergy Clin. Immunol.* 1986;77:537–543.

17 · Eosinophils and bronchial hyperresponsiveness in bronchial asthma

S.R. Durham

Asthma is characterized clinically by increased bronchial responsiveness to a wide variety of non-specific triggers and pathologically by the presence of eosinophils in blood [1], sputum [2], bronchoalveolar lavage fluid and in bronchial mucosal biopsies [3]. Even in mild asthmatics, the numbers of eosinophils in blood and bronchoalveolar lavage fluid are increased and correlate inversely with histamine PC_{20}; i.e. the higher the eosinophil count the more responsive the airways [1,3]. *In vitro* studies have shown that products from activated eosinophils may be important in the development of airway narrowing in asthma. For example, leukotriene (LT) C_4 is a potent mucus secretagogue and bronchoconstrictor. By use of immunofluorescent studies of autopsy material from asthma deaths, the eosinophil granule-derived major basic protein (MBP) has been localized to sites of bronchial epithelial damage [4]. Furthermore, MBP has been found in sputum from asthmatics in concentrations known to be toxic '*in vitro*' to human bronchial epithelium [2]. Although these observations do not imply a causal relationship, there appears to be a strong association between eosinophils and tissue damage in bronchial asthma.

The late asthmatic response which follows allergen inhalation challenge has been used as a clinical model in order to investigate the relationship between eosinophils and increased bronchial responsiveness in allergic asthma. Studies in animal models and in man have illustrated the IgE-dependency of allergen-induced late responses in the skin, nose and lung. The development of late responses at these different tissue sites is accompanied by an eosinophil-rich cellular infiltrate. Previous studies of human allergen-induced late asthmatic responses have shown increased bronchial responsiveness at 24 h after inhalation challenge and an increase in peripheral blood eosinophils at this timepoint [1,5]. Bronchoalveolar lavage fluid obtained at the time of development of late responses (6–7 h) similarly demonstrated increased eosinophil numbers and elevated eosinophil cationic protein (ECP) concentrations [6].

In view of these associations we have performed a randomized controlled clinical study involving allergen inhalation challenge in a group of asthmatic subjects. The aim was to examine the time-course and quantitative relationships amongst the development of late asthmatic responses, alterations in blood eosinophils and changes in airway histamine responsiveness. In order to assess a possible modulatory role for altered adrenal cortisol responsiveness, we also measured serum cortisol concentrations on both allergen and control days.

Fourteen atopic, non-smoking asthmatics were studied: eight subjects were female, six male. Baseline lung function (spirometry) was normal. There was a wide range of asthma severity as reflected by the baseline airway histamine responsiveness measurements which varied from moderately severely increased to within the normal non-asthmatic range (histamine PC_{20} 0.1–32 mg/ml). The subjects underwent two inhalation challenges with allergen and with allergen diluent (control day). The two challenges were performed in random order with an interval of 14 days.

Allergen and histamine inhalation challenge tests were performed as described. Eosinophil counts were assessed by an automated cell counter (Technicon H6000) and cortisol assayed by use of competitive radioimmunoassay. These measurements were performed before inhalation challenge (0930 h) and at 3 h after allergen (before the late response) and at 24, 48 h and 2 weeks (after the late response). The results after allergen were compared with corresponding measurements after the control challenge with allergen diluent.

On the control day, no changes in FEV_1 (within 10% of baseline) or histamine PC_{20} (within a twofold concentration difference) were observed after allergen challenge. A definite late asthmatic ($\geqslant$ 15% fall in FEV_1) was observed in eight of the 14 subjects. The development of a late response was associated with a greater than fourfold decrease in histamine PC_{20} at 3 h and 24 h after challenge. These changes in airway responsiveness preceded the late asthmatic response, occurred independently of changes in airway calibre and were highly correlated with the size of the subsequent late response [7].

On the control day we observed the normal diurnal increase in blood eosinophils (at 3–9 h after challenge) which is known to occur in both asthmatic and normal subjects. By contrast, after allergen challenge there was a relative fall in eosinophil counts when compared with the control day (mean difference -0.09×10^9/l, $p < 0.005$). By the following morning eosinophil counts had risen compared with the control ($+0.11\times10^9$) and this increase was even greater at 48 h ($+0.20\times10^9$) (Fig. 17.1). The magnitude of the changes in blood eosinophils at 9 h were highly correlated with the size of the late response ($r = 0.72, p < 0.01$). These changes also correlated strongly with the associated changes in airway histamine responsiveness at 3 h ($r = 0.55$, $p < 0.05$), 24 h ($r = 0.82, p < 0.0001$) and 48 h ($r = 0.84, p < 0.0001$). The secondary increase in blood eosinophils at 24 and 48 h did not correlate with either the late response or changes in responsiveness [8]. It seems likely that these delayed increases in eosinophils represent a bone marrow response following recruitment of eosinophils to the lung at the time of development of the late response.

These close associations suggest that the tissue events which underlie the late asthmatic response including eosinophil recruitment may occur when there is no airway obstruction, before the late response is clinically apparent.

In view of the potent inhibitory effects of corticosteroids on the late response [9], and experiments in dogs which showed that metyrapone pretreatment ('medical

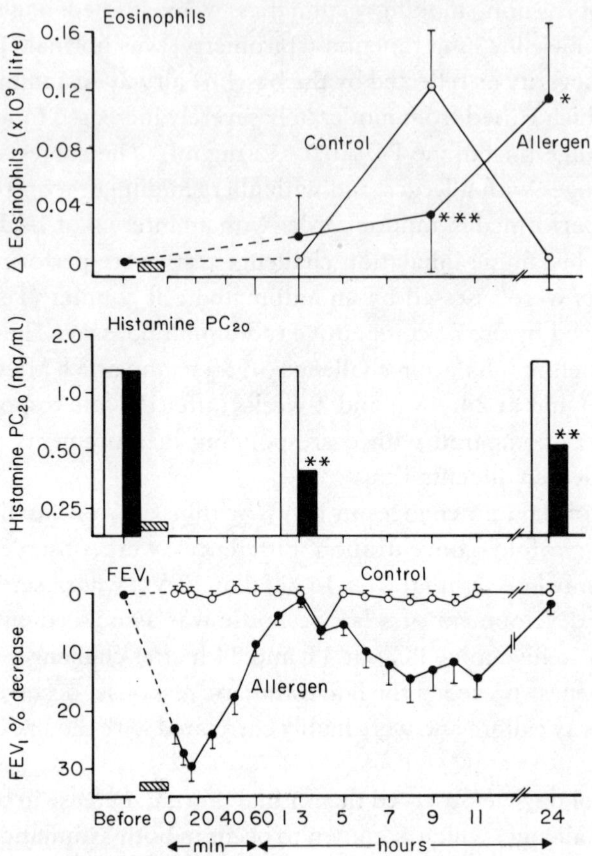

Fig. 17.1. The changes in peripheral eosinophil count ($\times 10^9$/l [mean ± SEM]), airway histamine responsivenes (mg/ml [geometric mean]) and FEV_1 (% change) following allergen and control inhalation challenge in 14 atopic asthmatic subjects ($* = p < 0.05$; $** = p < 0.01$; $*** = < 0.001$). There were no significant differences in baseline values for allergen and control days. (Reproduced from Cookson *et al. Am. Rev. Respir. Dis.* [8].

adrenalectomy') accentuated the late response [10], we postulated that altered adrenal responses after allergen challenge (increases in endogenous cortisol concentrations) might possibly represent a protective mechanism in the development of late responses. It turned out that a virtually identical normal diurnal decrease in blood cortisol concentrations was observed on both control and allergen days [11]. These changes had no relation to the presence or magnitude of the late response.

Finally we measured blood allergen-specific IgE during and up to 2 weeks after allergen-induced late responses. In contrast to the known seasonal increase in antibody concentrations no acute changes in IgE concentrations after the late response were observed.

Summary

In this randomized controlled study of allergen inhalation challenge we have shown that the late response was preceded by increases in airway histamine responsiveness and accompanied by a relative fall in blood eosinophils. Highly significant correlations amongst these three variables suggest that the tissue events which underlie the late response, including eosinophil recruitment, may begin when there is no overt airway obstruction and before the late response is clinically apparent. There were no acute changes in blood IgE antibody concentratons. Normal diurnal changes in blood cortisol concentrations were observed which did not support a role for altered adrenal responses, protective or otherwise, in the development of human late responses.

References

1 Durham SR, Kay AB. Eosinophils, bronchial hyperreactivity and late phase asthmatic reactions. *Clin. Allergy* 1985;**15**:411–418.

2 Frigas E, Loegering D, Solley G, Farrow G, Gleich GJ. Elevated levels of the eosinophil major basic protein in the sputum of patients with bronchial asthma. *Mayo Clin. Proc.* 1981;**56**:345–353.

3 Wardlaw AJ, Dunnette S, Gleich GJ, Collins JV, Kay AB. Eosinophils and mast cells in bronchoalveolar lavage in mild asthma: relationship to bronchial hyperreactivity. *Am. Rev. Respir. Dis.* 1988;**137**: 62–69.

4 Filley WV, Holley KE, Kephart GM, Gleich GJ. Identification by immunofluorescence of eosinophil granule major basic protein in lung tissues of patients with bronchial asthma. *Lancet* 1982;**ii**:11–16.

5 Booij-Nord H, de Vries K, Sluiter HJ, Orie NGM. Late bronchial obstructive reaction to experimental inhalation of house dust extract. *Clin. Allergy* 1972;**2**:43–61.

6 De Monchy JGR, Kauffman HF, Venge P, Koeter GH, Jansen HM, Sluiter HJ, De Vries K. Bronchoalveolar eosinophilia during allergen-induced late asthmatic reactions. *Am. Rev. Respir. Dis.* 1985;**131**:373–376.

7 Durham SR, Craddock CF, Cookson WOCM, Benson MK. Increases in airway histamine responsiveness precede allergen-induced late asthmatic responses. *J. Allergy Clin. Immunol.* 1988;**82**:764–770.

8 Cookson WOCM, Craddock CF, Benson MK, Durham SR. Falls in blood eosinophils parallel the late asthmatic response. *Am. Rev. Respir. Dis.* 1989;**139**:458–462.

9 Fabbri LM, Chiesura Corona P, Dal Vecchio L, Di Giacomo GR, Zocca E, De Marzo N, Maestrelli P, Mapp CE. Prednisone inhibits late asthmatic reactions and the associated increase in airway responsiveness induced by toluene diisocyanate in sensitized subjects. *Am. Rev. Respir. Dis.* 1985;**132**:1010–1014.

10 Sasaki H, Yanai M, Shimura S, Okayama H, Aikawa T, Sesaki T, Takishima T. Late asthmatic response to Ascaris antigen challenge in dogs pretreated with metyrapone. *Am. Rev. Respir. Dis.* 1987;**136**:1459–1465.

11 Durham SR, Keenan J, Cookson WOCM, Craddock CF, Benson MK. Diurnal variation in serum cortisol concentrations in asthmatic subjects after allergen inhalation. *Thorax* 1989;**44**:582–585.

18 · Pharmacology of eosinophils

P.J. Barnes, C. Kroegel, T. Yukawa, G. Dent and K.F. Chung

Introduction

Eosinophils may play a critical role in bronchial hyperresponsiveness and asthma [1], but the mechanisms involved in the selective recruitment and activation of eosinophils in the airways are still almost unknown. The mechanisms involved in modulation of eosinophil activation and secretion are also largely unexplored. This partly stems from the difficulties in obtaining adequate numbers of cells of significant purity for pharmacological and biochemical investigation. Furthermore, the process of purification may alter their responsiveness. Since the eosinophil may play a critical role in the pathophysiology of asthma it is important to understand in more detail the biochemical process involved in activation and secretion of these cells, the stimulus–response coupling mechanisms and the pharmacological means by which these processes may be modulated as a therapeutic approach to asthma. Even the effect of anti-asthma drugs in current clinical use on eosinophil function is hardly known. For these reasons we have embarked on a detailed study of the pharmacology of eosinophils.

Eosinophil preparation

We harvested eosinophils from guinea pig peritoneum by the method of Pincus [2]. Briefly, eosinophils were obtained from polymyxin B-treated male guinea pigs by weekly peritoneal lavage. The cells were purified using a discontinuous density gradient of isomolar Percoll solutions. Eosinophils with a purity of more than 95% and a viability of over 99% were obtained from fractions 3 to 5. The fractions were pooled and washed three times in Hanks balanced salt solution

Human eosinophils were prepared from blood taken from atopics, asthmatics or donors with hypereosinophilic syndrome. Eosinophils were purified from buffy coat cells on metrizamide [3] or Percoll density gradients [2]. Eosinophils with a purity of over 80% and a viability over 95% were collected from the 22, 23, and 24% metrizamide density interfaces.

Eosinophil activation

Eosinophils may be activated by a number of stimuli, including IgG [4], IgA [5], IgE [6], opsonized particles [7], the complement fragment C5a [8], and platelet-activating factor (PAF) [9], all of which stimulate specific surface receptors. In addition, calcium ionophore A23187, which translocates calcium into the cell, and phorbol esters such as phorbol myristate acetate (PMA), which directly activates protein kinase C, also stimulate eosinophil activation [10,11].

Eosinophils and PAF

Platelet-activating factor, a lipid mediator formed by the action of phospholipase A_2 on membrane alkylacyl phospholipids, may play an important role in asthma [12,13]. It is formed by several inflammatory cells which have been implicated in asthma, including macrophages [14] and eosinophils [15]. Indeed, eosinophils are the richest cellular source of PAF and hypodense eosinophils of asthmatic patients release particularly large amounts [15]. Platelet-activating factor has many properties which are relevant to asthma: it causes bronchoconstriction (indirectly, since it has no direct effect on airway smooth-muscle [16], is the most potent cause of airway microvascular leakage to date [17,18] and causes sustained increase in bronchial reactivity in several animal species (guinea pig, rabbit, dog, cat, sheep, primates) [19–22], including humans [23,24]. This latter property is what distinguishes PAF from other putative mediators of asthma [12] and may relate to the interaction between PAF and eosinophils.

Platelet-activating factor is potently chemotactic for human eosinophils *in vitro* and has a greater effect on eosinophils than on neutrophils [25,26]. It is also chemoattractant *in vivo* and causes eosinophil infiltration into the skin of atopic individuals [27], and into lungs of primates following both local [22,28] and systemic [29] administration. PAF also increased the adherence of eosinophils to cultured human umbilical vein endothelial cells at concentrations as low as 1 nM [30]. Platelet-activating factor enhances eosinophil-mediated killing of schistosomula opsonized with immune serum as a source of complement and IgG, or with purified specific IgE [31], and increases capacity of normodense eosinophils to bind IgE [32]. It also induces a shift in density from normodense to hypodense eosinophils *in vitro* [33]. Platelet-activating factor potently activates human eosinophils to secrete leukotriene (LT) C_4 [34], and to release granule contents, including eosinophil peroxidase (EPO), eosinophil cationic protein (ECP), beta-glucuronidase, alkaline and acid phosphatase and arylsulphatase B [9,35] (Fig. 18.1). This degranulation response to PAF is dose-related, non-cytotoxic and inhibited in a competitive manner by specific PAF-antagonists, such as the hetrazepine WEB 2086 or the ginkgolide BN 52021. Also the release of superoxide anions ($O_2^{\bar{\cdot}}$) from eosinophils is stimulated by PAF, although at 100-fold higher concentrations than needed for eliciting for chemotaxis or degranulation [35]. This suggests that different biochemical transduction mechanisms may be involved in the eosinophil activation by PAF [in preparation].

Platelet-activating factor receptors have been identified in eosinophils by direct binding studies with a labelled antagonist [^{3}H] WEB 2086 [36]. Labelled antagonists have proved to be far more useful than [^{3}H] PAF in studying binding sites, since the

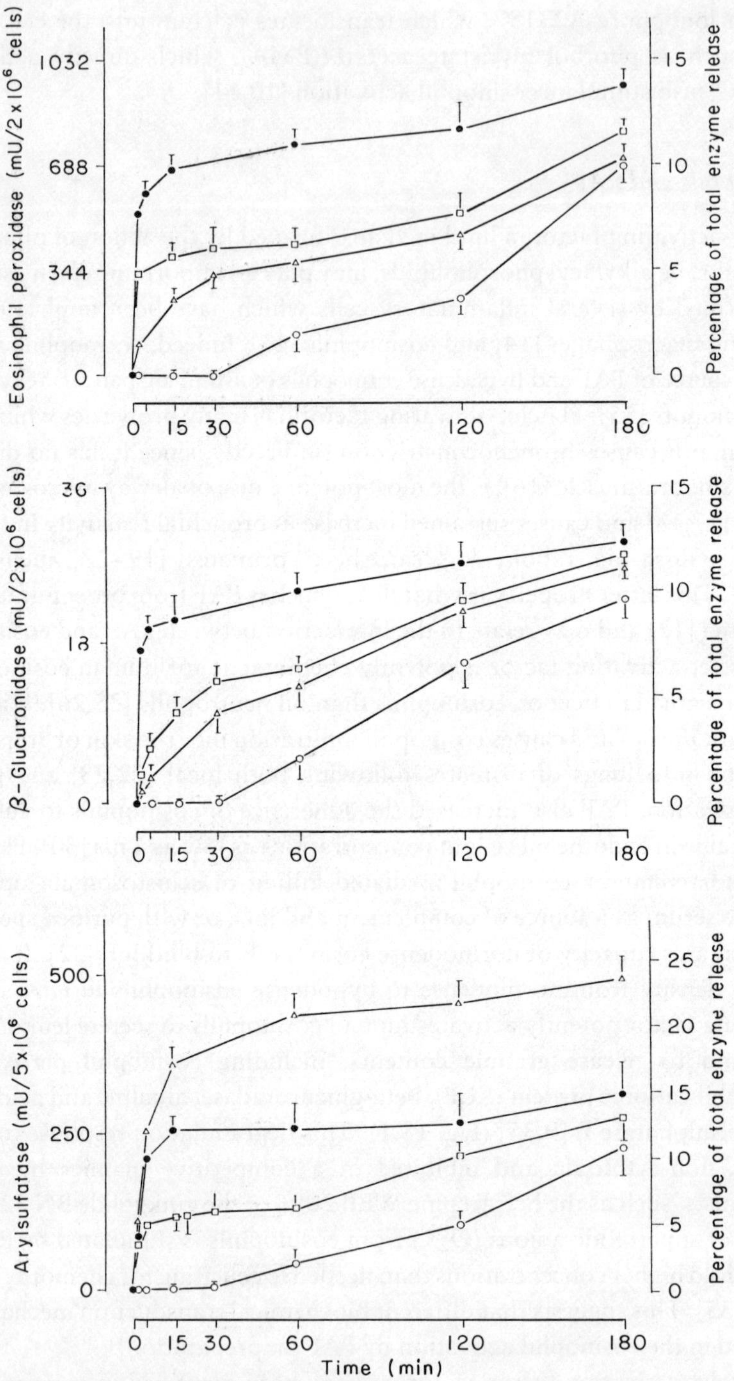

Fig. 18.1. The release of eosinophil peroxidase (A), β-glucuronidase (B), arylsulphatase (C) by human eosinophils stimulated with PAF (●) buffer control (○) [From 35].

problems of degradation and uptake of the ligand are avoided [37]. A high density of high affinity binding sites has been found in both guinea pig and human eosinophils (Fig. 18.2). The inhibitory potency of antagonists on specific binding is closely correlated with their potency in inhibiting PAF-mediated degranulation [36].

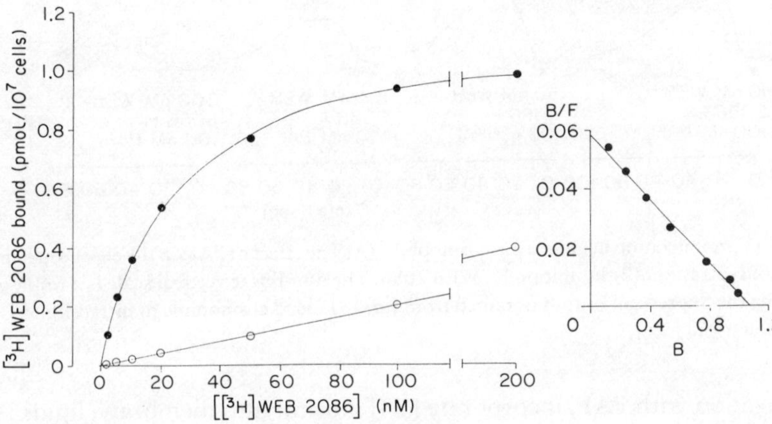

Fig. 18.2. The specific (●) and non-specific (○) binding of [^{3}H]WEB 2086 to human eosinophils. Inset: Scatchard plot of the same data.

The mechanism of stimulus–response coupling in eosinophils has been little investigated. Using PAF as an activating stimulus we have demonstrated a rapid and transitory rise in intracellular free calcium ion concentration ($[Ca^{2+}]_i$) in guinea pig eosinophils after exposure to PAF, using the fluorescent Ca^{2+} indicator dye fura-2 [38] (Fig. 18.3a). The response is blocked by WEB 2086 (Fig. 18.3b), and is dependent on the presence of extracellular Ca^{2+} as it is significantly inhibited by EGTA (which sequesters extracellular Ca^{2+}) or nickel ions (which inhibit Ca^{2+} entry by blocking the Ca^{2+} translocating pores) (Fig. 18.4). The Ca^{2+} influx is likely to occur through receptor-operated channels since the rise in $[Ca^{2+}]_i$ is not blocked by a voltage-dependent Ca^{2+} antagonist, nimodipine.

Optimal degranulation of inflammatory cells such as mast-cells or basophil leucocytes is dependent upon the presence of extracellular Ca^{2+} [39]. Similar results have been found in eosinophils for which it has been shown that PAF-induced degranulation was greatly diminished in the absence of Ca^{2+}. Hence, drugs which inhibit receptor-operated Ca^{2+} entry may therefore be effective in inhibiting eosinophil activation.

There is also a residual elevation of $[Ca^{2+}]_i$ after stimulation with PAF, even in the presence of Ni^{2+} ions or EGTA, indicating mobilization of free Ca^{2+} from intracellular stores. Such intracellular release of Ca^{2+} may be due to receptor-stimulated phosphoinositide (PI) hydrolysis as has been shown in other cells [40]. Eosinophils

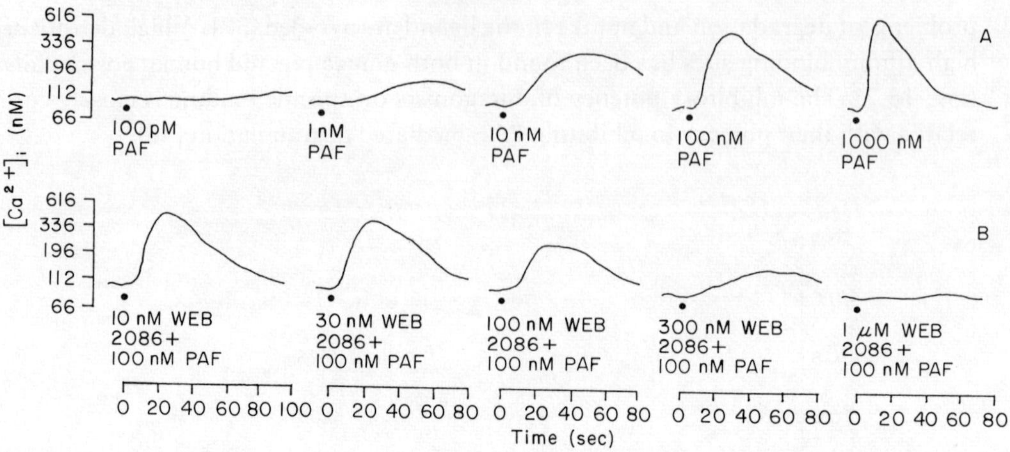

Fig. 18.3. Ca^{2+} mobilization in guinea pig eosinophils. (A) The effect of PAF on the elevation of intracellular free Ca^{2+} concentration. (B) Inhibition by WEB 2086. The non-linear vertical scale is a result of transforming the fluorescent output obtained from fura-2 loaded eosinophils to intracellular Ca^{2+} concentration (from [38]).

after activation with PAF, incorporate [^{3}H] inositol into membrane lipids [41], indicating PI hydrolysis. It has not yet proved possible, however, to separate the labelled inositol phosphates; this is presumably because of the presence of the highly charged eosinophil basic proteins which may absorb the labelled inositol phosphates and may interfere with the binding to the negatively charged stationary phase in ion-exchange chromatography.A competitive binding assay for IP3 looks to be a more promising approach [42].

The stimulus specific nature of PAF-elicited degranulation of human eosinophils

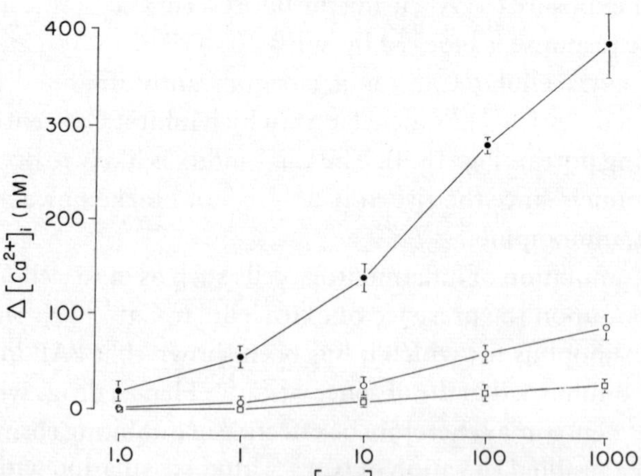

Fig. 18.4. The effect of extracellular Ca^{2+} (●), EGTA (○) and Ni^{2+} (□) on the rise in intracellular calcium concentration ($[Ca^{2+}]_i$) in guinea pig eosinophils (from [38]).

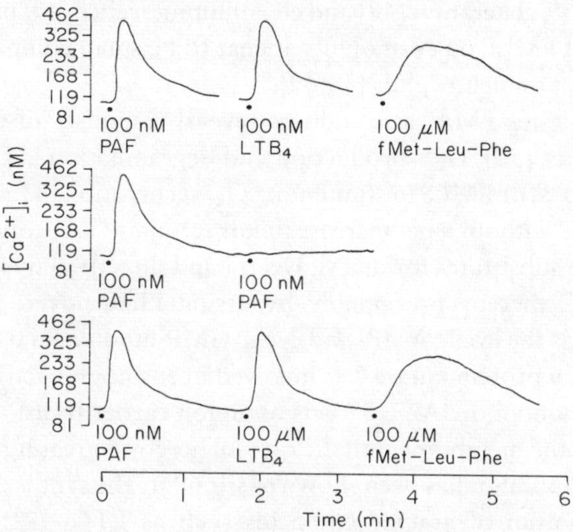

Fig. 18.5. Homologous desensitization of eosinophils stimulated with PAF, LTB_4 and FMLP (from [38]).

is further illustrated by the observation that cells pretreated with PAF rendered the eosinophils unresponsive to subsequent exposure to this stimulus, although the cells remain fully responsive to opsonized zymosan or calcium ionophore. In addition, after initial stimulation with PAF eosinophils do not respond with a further elevation of the cytoplasmic Ca^{2+} level whereas LTB_4 or the *N*-formylated chemotactic peptide formyl-methionine-leucine-phenylalanine (FMLP) produce a full response (Fig. 18.5). The attenuated capacity of eosinophils to release enzymes or increase $[Ca^{2+}]_i$ following a second application of the same stimulus is most likely caused by homologous desensitization. Stimulus desensitization has previously been demonstrated in neutrophils with PAF and other stimuli [43,44] but has not previously been reported in eosinophils.

Other stimuli

Several other stimuli are effective in stimulating eosinophils. Leukotriene B_4 induces eosinophil chemotaxis *in vitro* though its potency is weaker than the effect of PAF [25,26]. In addition, LTB_4 only produces a modest eosinophil accumulation after application in the skin of volunteers [45]. Also LTB_4 leads to a slight increase in the cytotoxic capacity of eosinophils for parasites [46]. However, LTB_4 causes a rapid increase of $[Ca^{2+}]$ in fura-2 loaded guinea pig eosinophils which is comparable with that induced by PAF [38].

The bacterial-derived peptide FMLP, also induces a rise in $[Ca^{2+}]_i$ in guinea pig eosinophils but the effect is weak and occurs at high concentrations of greater than 1 µM. The peptide FMLP, has also been shown to stimulate eosinophil LTC_4

secretion [47], $O_2^{\cdot-}$ generation [48] and chemiluminescence [49] in eosinophils. However, the effect of FMLP on eosinophils appear to be small compared with its potent stimulatory action on neutrophils [48,49].

The phorbol ester PMA, also induces several responses of eosinophils such as chemiluminescence [50], $O_2^{\cdot-}$ production and degranulation [35]. It is far more potent than PAF, LTB_4 or FMLP in stimulating $O_2^{\cdot-}$ generation [35,49]. However, PMA activated the cells without a net increase in intracellular Ca^{2+} concentration. Phorbyl myristate acetate substitutes for diacylglycerol and directly activates the intracellular protein kinase C thereby presumably bypassing PI turnover, measurable $[Ca^{2+}]_i$ changes, as well as the cyclic AMP- and cyclic GMP-modulated pathways [51]. These data suggest that a protein kinase C is involved in eosinophil activation.

The calcium ionophore A23187 acts as an ion carrier translocating extracellular calcium through the membrane into the cytosol hereby activating calcium-dependent enzymes. In eosinophils it has been shown to stimulate the synthesis of products of the oxidative metabolism of arachidonic acids such as LTC_4 [52], thromboxane B_2, prostaglandin E_2, prostaglandin $F_2\alpha$ [53] and PAF [15]. In addition, calcium ionophore A23187 induces a small respiratory burst [11], and secretes granular enzymes and proteins from human eosinophils [10,35].

Eosinophils express several receptors for immunoglobulins and complement factors on their surface and the occupation of these receptors by a specific ligand has been linked to eosinophil effector functions [1]. IgG, IgE, C3b-coated zymosan and C3b-coated sepharose have been shown to induce secretion of eosinophil granular proteins [54–56]. Eosinophils bind firmly to IgG bound on large surfaces which induces both generation of LTC_4 and synthesis of new membrane proteins [4]. C5a, which can be generated by different surfaces and antigen–antibody reactions via the classical and alternative pathway, has strong chemotactic activity for human eosinophils [57].

Stimulus–response coupling in eosinophils

Current evidence suggests that the biochemical transduction mechanism in eosinophils after stimulation with PAF is as follows: initially, an agonist binds to its specific receptor on the eosinophil membrane surface, which may be linked to a Ca^{2+} channel. The ligand receptor interaction presumably opens this channel and allows calcium entry into the cell. It may also activate a phosphodiesterase (phospholipase C) which breaks down inositol lipids in the plasma membrane to produce free arachidonic acid and diaglycerol [58]. The phospholipase C may further activate the turnover of phosphoinositides. The inositol lipid breakdown serves a dual-signalling role with production of two second messengers. The first metabolite, inositol 1,4,5-trisphosphate (IP_3), is responsible for eliciting mobilization of Ca^{2+} from intracellular sources [40], while the second 1,2-diaglycerol (DAG) primarily activates the phospholipid-dependent protein kinase C (PKC) [51]. In addition, PKC is activated by the increase in cytosolic free Ca^{2+} concentration. Calcium, either directly or after binding to calmodulin or other Ca^{2+}-binding proteins, may also activate a phospholipase A_2 [59,60], resulting in production and release of LTC_4 [61] and prostanoids [62]. In either case, activated PKC phosphorylates a set of target proteins which may include the phosphorylation of the receptor itself, the receptor-linked G-proteins or IP_3 phosphatase. This PKC-dependent phosphorylation, in turn, could explain the homologous or heterologous desensitization of eosinophils observed with various stimuli.

Effect of anti-asthmatic drugs

If the eosinophil plays a critical role in bronchial hyperresponsiveness and chronic asthma then drugs which prevent the accumulation and activation of eosinophils should be useful as anti-asthmatic therapy. The effects of the drugs in common clinical use for asthma treatment have not yet been studied in detail, however.

Beta-adrenoreceptor agonists

Beta-agonists are the most effective bronchodilators in current practice and act predominantly by relaxing airway smooth-muscle, but also by inhibiting mast-cell degranulation [63]. The β_2-agonist, salbutamol in therapeutically relevant concentrations has no significant effect on EPO release or O_2^- production from human or guinea pig eosinophils stimulated by PMA or opsonized zymosan, however [64]. This is surprising, since β_2-receptors are clearly demonstrable on eosinophils using direct binding with [^{125}I] iodopindolol (approximately 4000 receptors/cell) [65]. Furthermore, these receptors are coupled to adenylate cyclase, since β_2-agonists induce a rise in cyclic AMP, and an increase in protein kinase A activity.

The reason why β_2-receptor stimulation fails to modulate either degranulation or oxidative metabolism is not known, but it is consistent with the lack of effect of β-agonists in inhibiting either the late response to allergen [66,67], or the increased bronchial reactivity after allergen challenge [67], or in reducing bronchial hyperresponsiveness [68,69]. Perhaps salbutamol, as a partial agonist, is not effective as the increase in cyclic AMP is insufficient to inhibit degranulation. Longer acting β-agonists, such as salmeterol or a combination of a β-agonist with a phosphodiesterase (PDE) inhibitor which prevents the breakdown of intracellular cAMP, may be more effective. Another reason for the lack of effect of salbutamol on eosinophil function could be that desensitization of β-receptors may occur during the course of the experiments, as this has been observed in neutrophils [70].

Theophylline

Theophylline has a complex action on eosinophil activation [64]. At high concentrations

(10 mM) there is inhibition of $O_2^{\cdot-}$ release and this may be due to phosphodiesterase inhibition. However, at relevant clinical concentrations there is a significant enhancement of $O_2^{\cdot-}$ release (Fig. 18.6). This appears to be due to adenosine receptor antagonism, since it is also seen with 8-phenyltheophylline, which is a more potent adenosine antagonist (but does not have PDE-inhibitory activity). Adenosine reverses the potentiation of $O_2^{\cdot-}$ production by theophylline and the A_2-receptors are involved. This enhancement of $O_2^{\cdot-}$ release by theophylline is also seen with human neutrophils [71]. The clinical relevance of enhanced $O_2^{\cdot-}$ release by theophylline is not certain. Enprophylline, a methylxanthine which shares the bronchodilator and anti-asthma properties of theophylline, but does not inhibit adenosine receptors [72] might not be expected to have this effect.

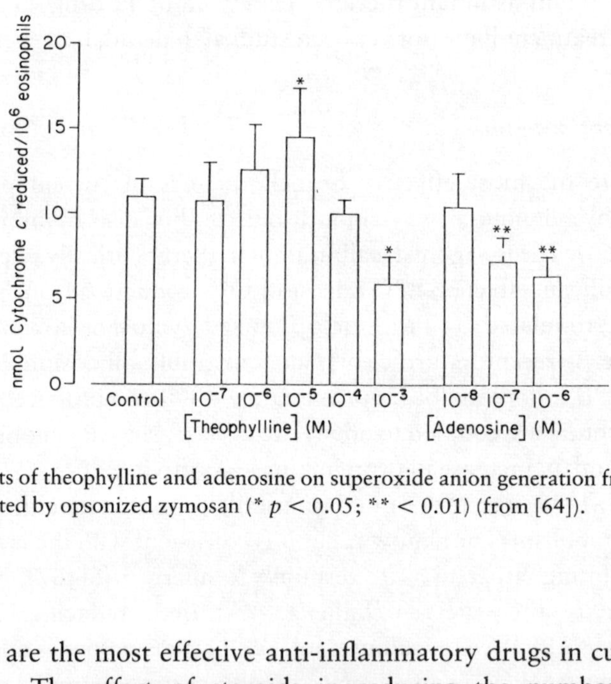

Fig. 18.6. The effects of theophylline and adenosine on superoxide anion generation from human eosinophils stimulated by opsonized zymosan (* $p < 0.05$; ** < 0.01) (from [64]).

Corticosteroids

Corticosteroids are the most effective anti-inflammatory drugs in current usage for asthma therapy. The effect of steroids in reducing the number of peripheral eosinophils is well known [73–75] which may be due to a decreased bone marrow release possibly as a result of a decreased production and release of eosinophil colony-stimulating factors by T-lymphocytes [76]. Steroids also inhibit eosinophil infiltration into tissues probably by inhibiting eosinophil chemotaxis [77]. Other effects of corticosteroids on eosinophils include prevention of Fc receptor expression [78].

Steroids may also have an inhibitory action on release of eosinophil products. Eosinophil cationic protein release by human eosinophils stimulated with complement-coated Sephadex beads is reduced by preincubating the cells with hydrocortisone for 30 min [79]. Furthermore, inhaled corticosteroids decrease the ECP serum concentration in asthmatic subjects [80] indicating an inhibitory effect of these drugs on eosinophil secretion. Preliminary *in vitro* studies using dexamethasone have suggested an inhibition of EPO and O_2^- release from eosinophils activated by opsonized zymosan and PMA [81]. Whether this effect is dependent on phospholipase A_2 inhibition or on some other action of steriods remains to be elucidated.

Future directions

Since PAF is the most potent chemotactic factor for human eosinophils to date, and also potently leads to the release of eosinophil basic proteins, application of specific PAF receptor antagonists, such as WEB 2086, may be used as a valuable tool in preventing eosinophil activation. Thus, PAF antagonists may prove beneficial for the therapeutic management of eosinophil-associated hypersensitivity diseases such as asthma.

Other approaches may aim at modulating key events in eosinophil cell activation. Drugs which inhibit receptor-operated Ca^{2+} influx could be of benefit and such drugs are under development. Eosinophils clearly have adenylate cyclase which may be activated by β-receptors, although beta-agonists, such as salbutamol, appear to be not effective in inhibiting the activation of the cells. However, adenosine, acting via A_2-receptors which also activates adenylate cyclase, does have a modest inhibitory effect. The action of other agonists which stimulate this enzyme, such as prostaglandin E_2 and I_2 and vasoactive intestinal peptide, must now be studied, together with cholera toxin which stimulates the stimulatory G-protein (Gs) and forskolin, which directly activate adenylate cyclase. Selective PDE inhibitors may also be effective, since high concentrations of theophylline inhibit release of oxygen metabolites. Several iso-enzymes of PDE are recognized [82] and it may be important to identify which is involved since selective PDE inhibitors are now available. Finally, the molecular basis for corticosteroid action on eosinophils also deserves further investigation, since drugs which mimic their effect such as phospholipase A_2 inhibitors could be of value.

Acknowledgements

The authors would like to thank the Medical Research Council and the Wellcome Trust for their support.

References

1 Gleich GJ, Adolphson CR. The eosinophilic leukocyte: structure and function. *Adv. Immunol.* 1986;39:177–253.
2 Pincus SH. Production of eosinophil-rich guinea pig peritoneal exudates. *Blood* 1978;52:127–135.
3 Fukuda T, Dunette SL, Reed CE, Ackerman SJ, Peter MS, Gleich GJ. Increased numbers of hypodense eosinophils in blood of patients with bronchial asthma. *Am. Rev. Respir. Dis.* 1985;132:981–985.

4 Thorne KJ, Free J, Franks D, Oliver RC. The mechanism of Fc-mediated interaction of eosinophils with immobilized immune complexes. II. Identification of two membrane proteins, modified by the interaction. *J. Cell Sci.* 1982;**56**:357–369.

5 Capron M, Tomassini M, Torpier G, Kusnierz JP, MacDonald S, Capron A. Selectivity of mediators released by eosinophils. *Int. Arch. Allergy Appl. Immunol.* 1989;**88**:54–58.

6 Capron M, Spiegelberg HL, Prin L, Bennich H, Butterworth AE, Pierce RJ, Ouaissi MA, Capron A. Role of IgE receptors in effector function of human eosinophils. *J. Imunol.* 1984;**132**:462–468.

7 Winquist I, Olofsson T, Olsson I. Mechanisms for eosinophil degranulation: release of eosinophil cationic protein. *Immunology* 1984;**51**:1–8.

8 De Simone C, Ferrari M, Pugnaloni L, Ferrarelli, Rumi C, Sorice F. Eosinophil-mediated cellular cytotoxicity induced by zymosan-activated serum. *Immunol. Letts.* 1986;**12**:37–41.

9 Kroegel C, Yukawa T, Dent G, Chung KF, Barnes PJ. Platelet activating factor induces eosinophil peroxidase release from human eosinophils. *Immunology* 1988;**64**:559–562.

10 Fukuda T, Ackerman SJ, Reed CE, Peters MS, Dunnette SL, Gleich GJ. Calcium ionophore A23187 calcium dependent cytolytic degranulation in human eosinophils. *J. Immunol.* 1985;**135**:1349–1356.

11 Yazdanbakhsh M, Eckmann CM, De Boer M, Roos D. Purification of eosinophils from normal human blood, preparation of eosinoplasts and characterization of their functional response to various stimuli. *Immunology* 1987;**60**:123–129.

12 Barnes PJ, Chung KF, Page CP. Inflammatory mediators and asthma. *Pharmacol. Rev.* 1988;**40**:49–84.

13 Barnes PJ, Chung KF, Page CP. Platelet activating factor as a mediator of allergic disease. *J. Allergy Clin. Immunol.* 1988;**81**:919–934.

14 Arnoux B, Duval D, Benveniste J. Release of platelet activating factor (PAF-acether) from alveolar macrophages by calcium ionophore A23187 and phagocytosis. *Eur. J. Clin. Invest.* 1980;**10**:437–441.

15 Lee T, Lenihan DJ, Malone B, Roddy LL, Wasserman SI. Increased biosynthesis of platelet-activating factor in activated human eosinophils. *J. Biol. Chem.* 1984;**259**:5526–5530.

16 Vargaftig BB, Lefort J, Chignard M, Benveniste J. Platelet activating factor induces a platelet-dependent bronchoconstriction unrelated to the formation of prostaglandin derivates. *Eur. J. Pharmacol.* 1980; **65**:185–192.

17 Evans TW, Chung KF, Rogers DF, Barnes PJ. Effect of platelet activating factor on airway vascular permeability: possible mechanisms. *J. Appl. Physiol.* 1987;**63**:479–489.

18 O'Donnell SR, Barrett CJK. Microvascular leakage to platelet activating factor in guinea pig trachea and bronchi. *Eur. J. Pharmacol.* 1987;**138**:385–396.

19 Mazzoni L, Morley J, Page CP, Sanjar S. Induction of airway hyperreactivity by platelet activating factor in guinea pig. *J. Physiol.* 1985;**365P**:P107.

20 Christman BW, Portes DK, King GA., Lefferts PL, Snapper JR. Synthetic platelet activating factor alters pulmonary haemodynamics, lung mechanics and lung fluid/solute exchange in awake sheep: role of platelets and granulocytes and effects of synthetic platelet activating factor on airway reactivity. *Am. Rev. Respir. Dis.* 1987;**133**:A174.

21 Chung KF, Aizawa H, Leikauf G, Ueki IF, Evans TW, Nadel JA. Airway hyperresponsiveness induced by platelet activating factor: role of thromboxane generation. *J. Pharmacol. Exp. Ther.* 1987;**236**:580–584.

22 Arnoux B̆, Dejean A, Page CP, Morley J, Benveniste J. Pulmonary effects of platelet activating factor in a primate are inhibited by ketotifen. *Am. Rev. Respir. Dis.* 1985;**131**:A2.

23 Cuss FM, Dixon CMS, Barnes PJ. Effects of inhaled platelet activating factor on pulmonary function and bronchial responsiveness in man. *Lancet* 1986;**ii**:189–192.

24 Rubin AE, Smith LJ, Patterson R. The bronchoconstrictor properties of platelet activating factor in humans. *Am. Rev. Respir. Dis.* 1987;**136**:1145–1151.

25 Wardlaw AJ, Moqbel R, Cromwell O, Kay AB. Platelet activating factor. A potent chemotactic and chemokinetic factor for human eosinophils. *J. Clin. Invest.* 1986;**78**:1701–1706.

26 Sigal CR, Valone FH, Holtzman MJ, Goetzl EJ. Preferential human eosinophil chemotactic activity of platelet activating factor (PAF) 1-O-alkyl-2-acetyl-*sn*-glycerol-3-phosphatidylcholine (AGEPC). *J. Clin. Immunol.* 1987;**7**:179–184.

27 Henocq E, Vargaftig BB. Skin eosinophilia in atopic patients. *J. Allergy Clin. Immunol.* 1988;**81**:691–695.

28 Henocq E, Vargaftig BB. Accumulation of eosinophils in response to intracutaneous PAF-acether and allergens in man. *Lancet* 1986;**ii**:1378–1379.

29 Lellouch-Tubiana A, Lefort J, Pirotzky E, Vargaftig BB, Pfister A. Ultra-structural evidence for extravascular platelet recruitment in the lung upon intravenous injection of platelet-activating factor (PAF-acether to guinea pigs). *Br. J. Exp. Pathol.* 1985;**66**:345–356.

30 Kimani G, Tonnesen MG, Henson PM. Stimulation of eosinophil adherence to human vascular endothelial cells *in vitro* by platelet-activating factor. *J. Immunol.* 1988;**140**:3161–3166.

31 Wardlaw AJ, Moqbel R, Kurihara K, Walsh G, Kay AB. Role of PAF-acether in leukocyte activation and chemotaxis. In *The Role of Platelet Activating Factor in Immune Disorders. New Trends in Lipid Research*, Vol. 2 (Ed. Braquet P.), Karger, Basel, 1988, pp. 691–695.

32 Walsh GM, Nagakura T, Iikura Y. Flow-cytometric analysis of increased IgE uptake by normal eosinophils following activation with PAF-acether and other inflammatory mediators. *Int. Arch. Allergy Appl. Immunol.* 1989;**88**:194–196.

33 Yukawa T, Kroegel C, Evans P, Fukuda T, Barnes PJ. Density heterogeneity of eosinophils: induction of hypodense eosinophils by platelet activating factor. *Immunology* 1989;**68**:140–143.

34 Bruynzeel PLB, Kok PTM, Haemelink ML, Kijne AM, Verhagen J. Platelet-activating factor induces leukotriene C_4 synthesis by purified human eosinophils. *Prostaglandins* 1987;**34**:205–214.

35 Kroegel C, Yukawa T, Dent G, Venge P, Chung KF, Barnes PJ. Stimulation of degranulation from human eosinophils by platelet activating factor. *J. Immunol.* 1989;**142**:3518–3526.

36 Ukena D, Kroegel C, Dent G, Yukawa T, Sybrecht G, Barnes PJ. PAF-receptors on eosinophils: identification with a novel ligand, [^{3}H) WEB 2086. *Biochem. Pharmacol.* 1989;**38**:1702–1705.

37 Dent G, Ukena D, Barnes PJ. PAF receptors. In *PAF and Human Disease* (Eds Barnes PJ, Page CP, Henson PM), Blackwell Scientific Publications, Oxford, 1989, pp. 58–81.

38 Kroegel C, Pleass R, Yukawa T, Chung KF, Westwick J, Barnes PJ. Characterization of platelet activating factor-induced elevation of cytosolic free calcium concentration in eosinophils. *FEBS Letts.* 1989;**243**:41–46.

39 Foreman JC, Hallett MB, Mongar JL. The relationship between histamine secretion and 45-calcium uptake by mast cells. *J. Physiol.* 1977;**271**:193–214.

40 Berridge MJ. Inositol trisphosphate and diaglycerol: two interacting second messengers. *Ann. Rev. Biochem.* 1987;**56**:159–193.

41 Kroegel C, Chilvers ER, Barnes PJ. Platelet activating factor (PAF) stimulates phosphoinositide (PI) metabolism in guinea pig eosinophils. *Clin. Sci.* 1989;**76**:45.

42 Kroegel C, Chilvers ER, Giembycz M, Challis RAJ, Barnes PJ. Signal transduction in eosinophils: temporal association of calcium mobilization and *D*-myo-inositol (1,4,5) triphosphate mass accumulation. *Am. Rev. Respir. Dis.* 1990 (in press).

43 Smith RJ, Bowman BJ, Iden SS, Kolaja GJ, Wiser SK. Biochemical, metabolic and morphologic characteristics of human neutrophil activation with pepstatin A. *Immunology* 1983;**49**:367–377.

44 Henson PM, Zanolari B, Schwartzman NA, Hong SR. Intracellular control of human neutrophil secretion. I.C5a-induced stimulus specific desensitization and the effects of cytochalasin B. *J. Immunol.* 1978;**121**:851–855.

45 Bisgaard H, Helquist S, Boudet L, Venge P, Dahl R, Sondergaard J. Chemotactic activity of LTB_4 in man. *Allergy* 1986;**41**:365–372.

46 Moqbel R, Kuhn SP, Goetzl EJ, Kay AB. Enhancement of neutrophil- and eosinophil-mediated complement-dependent killing of schistosomula of *Schistosoma mansoni in vitro* by leukotriene B_4. *Clin. Exp. Immunol.* 1983;**52**:519–527.

47 Shaw RJ, Walsh GM, Cromwell O, Moqbel R, Spry CJ, Kay AB. Activated human eosinophils generate SRS-A leukotrienes following IgG-dependent stimulation. *Nature* 1985;**316**:120–122.

48 Yazdanbakshsh M, Eckmann C, Koenderman L, Verhoeven AJ, Roos D. Eosinophils do respond to fMLP. *Blood* 1987;**70**:379–383.

49 Palmblad J, Gyllenhammer H, Lindgren JA, Malmsten CL. Effects of leukotrienes and f-Met-Leu-Phe

on oxidative metabolism of neutrophils and eosinophils. *J. Immunol.* 1984;**132**:3041–3045.

50 Shult PA, Grazaiano FM, Wallow IH, Busse WW. Comparison of superoxide generation and luminol-dependent chemiluminescence with eosinophils and neutrophils from normal individuals. *J. Lab. Clin. Med.* 1985;**106**:638–645.

51 Nishizuka Y. The role of protein kinase C in cell surface signal transduction and tumor promotion. *Nature* 1984;**308**:693–698.

52 Jorg A, Henderson WR, Murphy RC, Klebanoff SJ. Leukotriene generation by eosinophils. *J. Exp. Med.* 1982;**155**:390–402.

53 Foegh ML, Maddox YT, Ramwell P. Human peritoneal eosinophils and formation of arachidonate cyclooxygenase products. *Scand. J. Immunol.* 1986;**23**:599–603.

54 Khalife J, Capron M, Cesbron JY, Tai P-C, Taelman H, Prin L, Capron A. Role of specific IgE antibodies in peroxidase (EPO) release from human eosinophils. *J. Immunol.* 1986;**137**:1659–1564.

55 Okuda M, Takenaka T, Kawabori S, Ogami Y. Ultrastructural study of the specific granule of the human eosinophil. *J. Submicrosc. Cytol.* 1981;**13**:465–471.

56 Glaudert AM, Oliver RC, Thorne KJ. The interaction of human eosinophils and neutrophils with non-phagocytosable surfaces: a model for studying cell-mediated immunity in schistosomiasis. *Parasitology* 1980;**80**:525–537.

57 Ogawa H, Kunkel SL, Fantone JC, Ward PA. Digestion of the fifth component of complement by eosinophil lysosomal enzymes: production of eosinophil specific chemotactic activity. *Virchows Arch. Cell Pathol.* 1981;**38**:149–157.

58 Henderson WR, Chi EY, Jorg A, Klebanoff SJ. Horse eosinophil degranulation induced by the ionophore A23187. Ultrastructure and role of phospholipase A_2. *Am. J. Pathol.* 1983;**111**:341–349.

59. Matsumato T, Tao W, Sha'afi RI. Demonstration of calcium-dependent phospholipase A_2 activity in membrane preparation of rabbit neutrophils. Absence of activation by fMet-Leu-Phe, phorbol 12-myristate 13-acetate and A-kinase. *Biochem. J.* 1988;**250**:343–348.

60 Nishizuka Y. Studies and perspectives of protein kinase C. *Science* 1986;**233**:305–312.

61 Owen WF, Soberman RJ, Yoshimoto T, Sheffer AL, Lewis RA, Austen KF. Synthesis and release of leukotriene C_4 by human eosinophils. *J. Immunol.* 1987;**138**:532–538.

62 Morley J, Bray MA, Jones RW, Nugteren DH, van Dorp DA. Prostaglandin and thromboxane production by human and guinea pig macrophages and leukocytes. *Prostaglandins* 1979;**17**:730–746.

63 Barnes PJ, Dollery CT. Beta-adrenoreceptors in asthma and their response to agonists. In *Asthma: Physiology, Immunopharmacology and Treatment* (Eds Kay AB, Austen KF, Lichtenstein LM), Academic Press, New York, 1984; pp. 339–358.

64 Yukawa T, Kroegel C, Chanez P, Dent G, Ukena D, Chung KF, Barnes PJ. Effect of theophylline and adenosine on eosinophil function. *Am. Rev. Respir. Dis.* 1989;**140**:327–333.

65 Yukawa T, Ukena D, Chanez P, Dent G, Chung KF, Barnes PJ. Beta-adrenergic receptors on eosinophils: binding and functional studies. *Am. Rev. Respir. Dis.* 1990 (in press).

66 Hegart B, Pauwels R, von der Straeten M, Inhibitory effect of KWD 2131 terbutaline and DSCG on the immediate and late allergen-induced bronchoconstriction. *Allergy* 1981;**36**:115–122.

67 Cockroft DW, Murdock KY. Comparative effects of inhaled salbutamol, sodium cromoglycate and beclomethasone dipropionate on allergen-induced early asthmatic responses, late-asthmatic responses and increased bronchial responsiveness to histamine. *J. Allergy Clin. Immunol.* 1987;**79**:734–740.

68 Kraan J, Koeter GH, van der Mark TW, Sluiter HJ, de Vries K. Changes in bronchial hyperreactivity induced by 4 weeks of treatment with antiasthmatic drugs in patients with allergic asthma; a comparison between budesonide and terbutaline. *J. Allergy Clin. Immunol.* 1985;**76**:628–636.

69 Kerrebijn KF, van Essen-Zandvliet EEM, Neijens HJ. Effect of long-term treatment with inhaled corticosteroids and beta-agonists on the bronchial responsiveness in asthmatic children. *J. Allergy Clin. Immunol.* 1987;**79**:653–659.

70 Tecoma ES, Motulsky HJ, Traynor AE, Omann GM, Muller H, Sklar LA. Transient catecholamine modulation of neutrophil activation: Kinetic and intracellular aspects of isoproterenol action. *J. Leuk. Biol.* 1986;**40**:629–644.

71 Schrier DJ, Imre KM. The effects of adenosine agonists on human neutrophil function. *J. Immunol.* 1986;137:3284–3289.
72 Persson CGA. Development of safer xanthine drugs for the treatment of obstructive airway disease. *J. Allergy Clin. Immunol.* 1986;78:817–824.
73 Baigelman W, Chodosh S, Pizzuto D, Cupples LA. Sputum and blood eosinophils during corticosteroid treatment of acute exacerbations of asthma. *Am. J. Med.* 1983;75:929–936.
74 Anderson V. Autoradiographic studies of eosinophil kinetics: effects of cortisol. *Cell Tissue Kinet.* 1969;2:139–146.
75 Sabag N, Castrillon MA, Tchernitchin A. Cortisol-induced migration of eosinophil leukocytes to lymphoid organs. *Experientia* 1978;**34**:666–667.
76 Slavick FT, Abboud CN, Brennan JK, Lichtman MA. Modulation of *in vitro* eosinophil progenitors by hydrocortisone: role of accessory cells and interleukins. *Blood* 1985;**66**:1072–1079.
77 Hudson G. Eosinophil granulocyte reactions. In *Bone Marrow Reactions* (Ed. Yoffey JM.), William & Wilkins, Baltimore, 1966, pp. 86–99.
78 Oliver RC, Glauert AM, Thorne KJI. Mechanisms of Fc-mediated interaction of eosinophils with immobilized immune complexes. I. Effects of inhibitors and activators of eosinophil function. *J. Cell Sci.* 1982;**56**:337–356.
79 Winqvist I, Olofsson T, Olsson I. Mechanism for eosinophil degranulation; release of the eosinophil cationic protein. *Immunology* 1984;**51**:1–8.
80 Dahl R, Venge P, Fredens K. Eosinophils. In *Asthma: Basic Mechanisms and Clinical Management* (Eds Barnes PJ, Rodger IW, Thomson NC.), Academic Press, London, 1988, pp. 115–129.
81 Yukawa T, Dent G, Kroegel C, Evans P, Barnes PJ, Chung KF. Inhibition of human and guinea pig eosinophil function *in vitro* by corticosteroids. *Thorax* 1989;**44**:883.
82 Bryson SE, Rodger IW. Effects of phosphodiesterase inhibitors on normal and chemically-skinned guinea pig isolated airway smooth muscle. *Br. J. Pharmacol.* 1987;**92**:673–681.

Index